Voices of Lung Cancer

The Healing Companion:
Stories for Courage,
Comfort and Strength

Edited by

The Healing Project

www.thehealingproject.org

"Voices Of" Series Book No. 1

LaChancepublishing

LACHANCE PUBLISHING • NEW YORK
www.lachancepublishing.com

Library of Congress Control Number: 2006936115

Publisher: LaChance Publishing LLC
            120 Bond Street
            Brooklyn, NY 11201
            www.lachancepublishing.com

All things have a beginning, although sometimes the journey from beginning to end is not always so clear and straightforward. While work on *Voices Of* began just two years ago, truth be told, the seeds were planted long ago by beloved sources. This book is dedicated to Jennie, Larry and Denise, who in the face of all things good and bad extended courage and support in excess. And especially to Richard, who taught us by the way he lived his life that anything is possible given enough time, hard work and love.

Contents

Part I: MESSAGES

Part II: INSPIRATION

Part III: TAKING CHARGE

Part IV: RECONNECTING

Part V: LEARNING

Part VI: PASSINGS

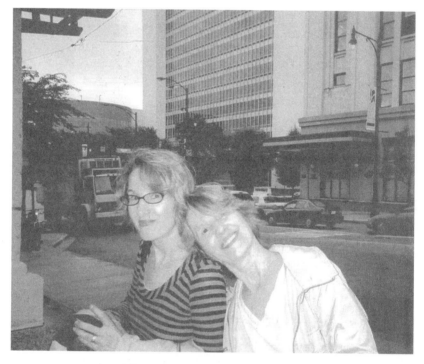

Denise and Debra LaChance

Introduction

~~

I wanted to ask the people around me, "Would you please raise your hand if you feel as isolated as I do?"

Walking the busy streets of Manhattan on a beautiful sunny day, I was surrounded by people but I'd never felt so alone. Just minutes before, my doctors had broken the news to me that I had a particularly aggressive form of breast cancer.

Since moving to New York from a small town in Rhode Island, I'd had my share of ups and downs but had always risen to the challenges that living and working in New York can bring. But on this summer afternoon, I felt as if the world was suddenly rushing past me while I moved in slow motion along the crowded sidewalk, wondering how I was going to tell my twin sister Denise that I had cancer.

My sister and I are as close as only twins can be: she is my best friend, my greatest support, my closest confidante. She was always at my side as I built successful businesses in fashion, technology, and real estate. We had faced challenges together in the past, but cancer was new territory. I thought that telling my loved ones would be worse than hearing it myself.

But with a life of love and support behind us and uncertainty ahead, Denise and I did what we had always done when faced with trouble: we cried and then we got to work. There was much to do and a short amount of time in which to do it: specialists to consult; doctors to interview; treatment plans to decide upon; hospitals to find. All the while the clock was ticking, urging me forward.

We made progress finding out about the disease and how best to treat it. But I could not shake the sense of aloneness I felt from the moment I received my diagnosis. I needed to hear from other people who had gone through what I had, who truly understood what it meant and who might be able to help. I wasn't ready for a regular support group and with surgery and treatment looming, I simply didn't have the time. But I am an avid reader and I assumed that finding the personal stories of those who had gone through this ordeal before me would be relatively easy. But finding what I needed turned out to be hard: where were the *real people* to talk to? Where were the books that weren't just about the science of the disease but about the emotional turmoil, the impact of the disease on every aspect of one's life?

There was one book gave me great comfort, *Just Get Me Through This* by Deborah Cohen and Robert A. Gelfand. It was a personal, rather than a clinical story and it sparked in me a desire for more stories that get to the heart of the emotional experience, that help the reader through it. In my limited time talking with other breast cancer patients, I knew there were countless others out there who needed to tell their stories—and to hear the stories of others as well. I decided that part of my own, ongoing healing process would be to find a way to bring people like me together, to create some kind of connection, where these real stories could be shared.

But first I had to find the doctors who would make the physical healing possible. As Denise and I did the research about the disease and its treatment, one doctor's name kept repeating: Dr. Alexander Swistel, Director of the Weill Cornell Breast Center at Weill Medical College at Cornell University. After meeting with him I knew he would be the one. It was scary enough to go through this at all, let alone do it with a surgeon who didn't make me feel as comfortable as possible. Dr. Swistel put me at my ease, gave me confidence and made me feel that I was in good hands.

I also felt instant rapport with my oncologist, Ellen Gold. Dr. Gold was frank and honest, while leaving me room to express my concerns. For many cancer patients, between diagnosis and the start of treatment there's little time to bring up feelings, much less have them addressed. The whole process moves so quickly the patient can feel as if she's being run through a healthcare assembly line with no chance to even firmly attach names to the faces of the many medical professionals responsible for her care. Dr. Gold always made me feel that there was time.

At first, what got me through that process were the little lies I told myself that allowed me to believe I would get through this. I'd seen my pathology report and I devoured all the literature on the disease, selecting the information that put the most positive "spin" on my condition. There's so much information out there, so many statistics, reports and findings that I could always find something to latch onto that would allow me to continually push the scariest possibilities away.

But the initial pathology report was wrong. The corrected report I received soon after the first indicated the highest presence of Her-2 (human epidermal growth factor receptor), which results in significantly worse survival rates in patients because its presence can lead to an intense proliferation of cancer cells. Time stood still for me as I read this new report and in that stillness I finally felt the full impact of my diagnosis. It was then that denial stopped working: I knew I'd need chemotherapy. Like so many women, the thought of losing my hair to chemotherapy brought it all crashing home, and as it is with many other patients, it was my turning point. Hitting that hard wall of reality, the time had come to finally face it and fight... or not.

I chose to fight, and in making that choice my vision of community crystallized and *The Healing Project* was born. I'd already realized that having access to the real stories of real people would make the journey through breast cancer much easier to endure. My thoughts kept returning to that walk through Manhattan after I'd heard my diagnosis and that feeling I had of terrible loneliness. As sympathetic as friends and loved ones could be, I felt that no one could truly understand this journey except those who had walked in the same shoes. As my surgery drew closer, I became convinced that getting and giving courage, comfort, and strength were as important as good medical care and I became determined to help build a community for people like me who were undergoing the terribly isolating experience of dealing with a life-threatening disease. This would be *The Healing Project*'s mission: to become a bridge across which people can make those all-important emotional connections. And talk about emotional connection: when I told Dr. Gold about the project, her eyes actually welled up with tears.

The hardest moment I had was when I had to leave Denise behind at the door of the operating room. But Doctor Swistel actually came out and walked me in. What a blessing. He even called me from his vacation later to check up on how I was doing.I had a second operation after the first failed to clear the margins of my cancer, then sixteen weeks of chemotherapy every two weeks followed by radiation, every day for seven weeks. I lost my hair in the first three weeks. I didn't want to watch as it came out in clumps until it was all gone, so I went out and had it shaved off. And with this reality of the disease giving me a yardstick to measure my priorities, I felt fine about it: it gave me another task I could do for myself, rather than just sitting around and waiting. Staying as active, and as proactive, as possible was very important to me. Throughout the ordeal I didn't stop working and went about my life with as much zeal as my varying energies would allow.

Following radiation, Dr. Gold told me that my biomarkers indicated I was a candidate for the new drug Herceptin which targets Her-2 and which had shown remarkable success in patients with aggressive breast cancer. Since the first round of chemo had caused damage to my heart and heart damage is also a possible side effect of of the use of Herceptin, I needed to be monitored during the treatments. If good things come in threes, my cardiologist, Doctor Allison Spatz, was my third miraculous doctor. She paid close attention to my case and when she went off my insurance plan in the middle of my treatment, she actually refused to take payment for her work! I ultimately took Herceptin for a year with good results.

During chemotherapy, Dr. Gold also encouraged my interest in exploring alternative and complementary treatment, including herbal mixtures and vitamin supplements. This, in combination with traditional medicine, did indeed help me. I know some people don't believe in the holistic approach, but for me I want to believe it worked. My immune system was pumped up when it should have been down and I didn't get the flu like so many other people in New York that season. To me, that's an important point about dealing with cancer: it comes down to what you choose to believe. There are so many people with so many opinions and there are so many variables to consider. Ultimately, you have to do what's right for yourself, realize that you're not as alone as you might feel, and seek out the people who know best what it's like to be you.

And those are the people I want to help me build *The Healing Project* community. In addition to my daily work during my treatments and during my second round of chemotherapy, I began to develop *The Healing Project* as a place where people can contribute funds for research, time for connecting with and mentoring others and, most of all, a place to share their stories. Since then, *The Healing Project* has been collecting stories by those touched by breast cancer and other diseases for books like this one: books that inspire and inform for the road ahead and impart a sense of community for those caught up in dealing with the moment. When you're sick or afraid, it's a godsend to know that there are others who understand. The stories we received from all over the country and beyond gave me exactly what I thought had been missing: personal stories that are a companion for patients, their friends, and families, an oasis where they can find strength in shared experiences.

In addition to the books, we're also working on other initiatives through *The Healing Project*, including "Voices Who Care," a virtual support group which will allow patients, family, and friends to connect with others online in real time. I don't want anyone to have to feel the way I did that day of my diagnosis when I was walking through the city alone and afraid. There's so much strength in others—you just have to find them. I think of the people who were here for me: Denise, Doctor Gold, Doctor Swistel, and Doctor Spatz and I realize how fortunate I was to have people who were willing to give of themselves and their time. The healing begins with giving to others.

So *The Healing Project* is part of my own healing, a signpost on my road ahead. And looking ahead, friends ask me if I consider myself cancer free. I choose not to. "The Big C" gives me something tangible with which I can measure my life. I guess I can't help being an entrepreneur, so I see the experience of cancer as an opportunity, with its own list of "Big C's":

To show Courage in the face of so much challenge.

To accept Caring as it comes.

To take Comfort from others.

To know it is OK to Complain.

To stay Connected with those you love.

To share with the Community your smiles, tears and fears.

To be Constant in your ability to rise above but never feel guilty when you can't.

To build Character for when you come out on the other side.

To Create kinship with others not as lucky as you.

To say I Can.

To say I Cannot.

To opt for Plan "C" if you must.

To take Control of your diagnosis and become your own advocate.

To believe in a Cure, if only for your heart.

To make Choices that you can live or die with.

Finally, with cancer you have to be ready to chart a new Course, for the rest of your life, no matter what the outcome. And it helps to see that others are busy charting their own courses along with you. That's what these stories are all about. Reading these amazing contributions to *The Voices Of* series convinces me that I don't really have a uniquely remarkable story at all.

The truth is *everyone* does.

Debra LaChance is the creator and founder of The Healing Project.

The Healing Project

Individuals diagnosed with life threatening or chronic, debilitating illnesses face countless physical, emotional, psychological, social, spiritual, and financial challenges during their treatment and throughout their lives. Emotional and social support from family members, friends, and the community at large is essential to their successful recovery and their quality of life; access to accurate and current information about their illnesses enables patients and their caretakers to make informed decisions about treatment and post-treatment care. Founded in 2005 by Debra LaChance, *The Healing Project* is dedicated to promoting the health and well being of these individuals, developing resources to enhance their quality of life and supporting the family members and friends who care for them. The Healing Project creates ways in which individuals can share their stories while providing access to current information about their illnesses. For more information about *The Healing Project* and its programs, please visit our website: www.thehealingproject .org.

Acknowledgments

This book would not have been possible had it not been for the selfless dedication of many, many people giving freely of their valuable time and expertise. We'd particularly like to thank Amy Shore, Barbara Jeanne Fischer, Richard Day Gore and Ann Marr for their work in reviewing all of the countless essays we received and for their editing prowess; Larry Bennett for steering the ship early on; Lisa LaChance for her assistance with almost every aspect of the project; Theresa Russell for her unending efforts to reach out to the many people and organizations making so many contributions to this book; Justin Cho for volunteering his time and sweating all the details; Melissa Marr for her astounding, ground-up organizational talents; Drs. Reed Phillips and Michael Vincent Smith for their extraordinary medical expertise; Susan C. Mantel and Diane Blum for their interest, advice and support; Victor Starsia, for setting the bar high and making sure we all made it over; to Gail Matthews and Dr. Marvelle Colby, for their boundless generosity with so many things; and to the many, many people who submitted stories to us, for their courage, their generosity and their humanity.

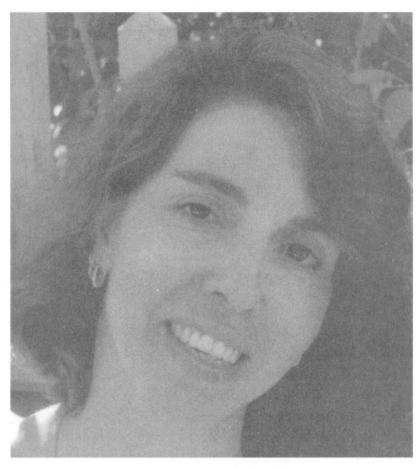

Joan Scarangello, page 51

Part I
MESSAGES

What do we live for if not to make life less difficult for each other?

—*George Eliot*

Cancer*Care*
Diane Blum

Lung cancer is the most common cause of cancer death in the United States. Yet in 2000, a media survey by Cancer*Care* confirmed that lung cancer was receiving far less coverage in print, broadcast, and online news than breast, colon and prostate cancers even though it claims more lives each year than these three other cancers combined. The survey also found that there were few celebrity spokespersons for lung cancer, few events to raise awareness, few first-person accounts about what it is like to live with the illness and little attention to progress being made in detection or treatment. Moreover, what little coverage there was of lung cancer was overshadowed by tobacco-related issues, something that both reflected and perpetuated a "blame the victim" attitude.

That same year, Cancer*Care* launched Lung Cancer Awareness Week, a national campaign focused on disseminating information, erasing the stigma associated with lung cancer and increasing the overall understanding of the risks as well as the options available to patients diagnosed with this illness. Too often we saw how stigmatization led to isolation for people coping with lung cancer and frequently prevented them from understanding their treatment options. No matter what the cause of cancer—and keep in mind that a high percentage of people diagnosed with lung cancer gave up smoking a long time ago—no one deserves to get it and everyone who does deserves to get the best possible treatment and care. They have a right to learn about resources available to them and their families, to ask for second opinions, to get help and to have hope.

It's been more than half a decade since CancerCare's media survey and the founding of Lung Cancer Awareness Week. In that time, we as a society have made great strides in providing comfort and support to people with lung cancer and their loved ones. This progress is the result of tireless efforts of many organizations and individuals dedicated to raising awareness and advocating for people with lung cancer. The media, too, is becoming a voice for this group. Newspapers and magazines have increased coverage of lung cancer issues, are less likely to focus solely on smoking and tobacco when reporting on it and offer more information on supportive care, clinical trials and research advances. As executive director of CancerCare, I've witnessed first-hand what the power of the media's attention can do to elevate national awareness and change public perception, and I have been fortunate to participate in the development of programs and services that share these goals.

In my position, I've been asked to support many publications aimed at people with cancer as well as books about cancer for the general public. I don't always take writers and publishers up on their offers, but once in a while a book comes along that not only really moves me, but also complements the mission of CancerCare to provide help and hope for all people affected by cancer. *Voices of Lung Cancer* is one such book. It is a rare tapestry of stories that illustrates the depth and variation of the lung cancer experience. The stories are written by people with cancer and by their spouses and partners, sons and daughters, brothers and sisters, caregivers and friends. The separate accounts weave together precious memories of life before cancer and tales of courage and strength in the face of diagnosis and treatment. Most of all, they celebrate life and illustrate the love and support that carry us through adversity and give meaning to our lives.

If you or someone you love has lung cancer, always remember that there are others going through similar experiences that can provide inspiration and hope. These individuals, as well as many cancer organizations can offer valuable insight and information on practical issues such as treatment options, managing changes in your daily life caused by cancer, and caring for the needs of your family at this time. I hope that *Voices of Lung Cancer* gives you comfort and reminds you that you are not alone in fighting this illness.

Diane Blum is the Executive Director of Cancer*Care*, a national nonprofit organization that since 1944 has provided free, professional counseling, education, financial assistance and practical help to millions of people affected by cancer. Co-founder of the National Alliance of Breast Cancer Organizations, Ms. Blum is a founder of National Breast Cancer Awareness Month and serves as Editor-in-Chief of People Living with Cancer, the patient education website of the American Society of Clinical Oncology (ASCO). Ms. Blum is the recipient of the Lifetime Achievement Award from the Board of Sponsors of National Breast Cancer Awareness Month, the Special Recognition Award from the National Coalition for Cancer Survivorship, the Republic Bank Breast Cancer Research Foundation Award and the Special Recognition Award of the American Society of Clinical Oncology.

Joan's Legacy
Susan C. Mantel

I come from one of those families that seem to be disproportionately affected by cancer—of all kinds, and with varying outcomes. I mention this because the prevalence of cancer in my life was a fact I only fully noted two years ago, shortly after I began working for Joan's Legacy: The Joan Scarangello Foundation to Conquer Lung Cancer.

I was astonished that before joining Joan's Legacy, I knew so little about lung cancer, despite having had two uncles who were afflicted with it. The reality was that my family, like too many other families, did not have anyone with whom to share its experience, since 10 and 15 years ago people rarely spoke of their lung cancer. So in our isolation, we assumed that our experience was somehow unique, and we were left to make sense of it on our own, for better or worse.

Equally amazing to me is that Joan was one of more than 20,000 "never smokers," 80% of whom are women, who get lung cancer each year. In fact, despite the widespread perception that lung cancer is a "smoker's disease," more than 60% of patients diagnosed with lung cancer either never smoked or quit many years earlier. Although no one will claim smoking is good for you, the point is that smoking prevention and cessation programs will not cure lung cancer. Only research into early diagnosis and successful treatment will do that.

To date, federal funding for lung cancer research has been woefully inadequate when compared to the amount of funding allocated for research into other forms of cancer. Currently, funding for lung cancer research is only $1,829 per lung cancer death, compared to $23,474 for breast cancer and $14,360 for prostate cancer, both of which have early detection programs and highly successful treatments. This disparity highlights both lung cancer's lack of progress and the real impact that can be made with significant funding of research. This lack of attention to finding answers for those already affected by lung cancer inspired the brave founders of Joan's Legacy to undertake this huge challenge.

Now every day at Joan's Legacy, I am reminded that millions of other families have been affected by lung cancer as well, with about 164,000 new diagnoses each year. And I am inspired by the courage and wisdom of the many patients and families that I have the privilege of meeting every day.

No one deserves cancer, but everyone deserves support and love as they fight this challenging disease. All of us at Joan's Legacy are dedicated to funding research into earlier diagnosis and more effective treatment for lung cancer. We salute Debra LaChance and all who have shared their stories and are dedicated to making the voices of lung cancer heard.

Joan's Legacy: the Joan Scarangello Foundation to Conquer Lung Cancer is a unique non-profit organization committed to fighting lung cancer by funding innovative research and by focusing greater attention on the world's leading cancer killer.

Joan's Legacy is named for Joan Scarangello McNeive, a gifted writer, life-long New Yorker and nonsmoker who died at age 47 in 2001 after a valiant nine-month fight with lung cancer. The organization was founded by her family and many friends in response to the lack of available treatments for lung cancer and the lack of research funding by private, charitable, or government sources. In its first five years, Joan's Legacy has become a leading resource in the search for new treatments and a cure for lung cancer.

In its fifth year, Joan's Legacy will have awarded more than $2,000,000 in research grants to the finest cancer centers in the United States and will have helped raise awareness of lung cancer throughout the country. The first nonprofit in the U.S. to specifically identify inequities in research funding and cultivate lung cancer research with a special focus on non-tobacco-related issues in lung cancer, Joan's Legacy has quickly become recognized as the "venture capital fund" for lung cancer research in the U.S.

Susan C. Mantel is the Executive Director of Joan's Legacy, putting into action its development and growth initiatives and developing collaborations with like-minded organizations across the country to achieve the common goal of finding a cure for a disease that will take the lives of over 160,000 Americans this year.

Lung Cancer Alliance
Laurie Fenton

Lung Cancer Alliance (LCA) is the only national non-profit organization dedicated solely to patient support and advocacy for people living with lung cancer and those at risk for the disease. LCA
is committed to leading the movement to reverse decades of
stigma and neglect by empowering those with or at risk for the
disease, elevating awareness and changing health policy.

For too long, people and organizations with the power to determine health care policy have allowed lung cancer research and
early detection to remain under funded. Even more shocking is the
underlying but seldom openly discussed excuse: "Why spend public health dollars when they did it to themselves. Funding smoking
cessation programs will end lung cancer."

Getting the truth out to the public is the first challenge. Yes, smoking cessation is critical and we fully support programs that can
effectively help people break the addiction. But how many know
that over 60% of all new lung cancer cases are being diagnosed in
people who never smoked, or in those who quit, many of them
decades ago? Is the public even aware of the building epidemic of
lung cancer diagnoses in non-smoking women? Why is the public
health establishment not educating the public about the importance of early detection and specifically about rapidly advancing

CT scan technology that has been proven successful in diagnosing lung cancer at an early stage, when life-saving treatments can be carried out?

The stigma of smoking and the low number of survivors have been barriers to building a grass roots movement for change. Until now. The LCA motto says it all: No more excuses. No more lung cancer.

The more helping hands and voices we can marshal, the more effective our call for change will be. Every voice counts. We thank The Healing Project for giving those affected by lung cancer another avenue for being heard. *Voices of Lung Cancer* is their stories and in the end it is they who will change public health policy and make lung cancer a curable rather than lethal disease.

Laurie Fenton manages the strategic direction of Lung Cancer Alliance. As President, Laurie oversees the creation and implementation of the Alliance's public policy agenda and national grassroots network and the design, delivery and evaluation of quality education, support, outreach and volunteer programs to stakeholders. Laurie is Lung Cancer Alliance's primary liaison to community and government leaders, collaborating agencies, stakeholders, lung cancer care professionals and other strategic alliances.

I Miss My Friends

S. Epatha Merkerson

I'm one of five children in my family. We all smoked cigarettes. Not by example (my mother was never a smoker), but because that's what you did when we were growing up. You could smoke anywhere and advertising for smoking could be found everywhere: in the movies, magazines and television commercials. I smoked cigarettes for 23 years but quit in February of 1994, about three years after one of my sisters was diagnosed with lung cancer. Debbie is a lung cancer survivor because of a chance trip to the doctor. She thought she had bronchitis. Early detection saved my sister's life.

Yvette Hawkins and Billie Neal were two of my best friends. They were young, intelligent and vibrant women. They were funny and sensitive and creative. Yvette and Billie both died of lung cancer. By the time each of them had been diagnosed, the cancer had metastasized and they had only enough time to put their affairs in order. I was with Billie two days before she passed away and I was with Yvette when she took her last breath. I'd never seen anyone die before.

After my friends passed away, I began to learn more about lung cancer through organizations like the Campaign for Tobacco Free Kids and CancerCare. I became angry. There's so much to be done in the fight against lung cancer, first and foremost removing the stigma that comes with the disease: now we all know one does not have to smoke to get it. If information had been disseminated, if funding had been allocated for lung cancer research and tools for early detection years ago, my friends might still be alive today.

I'm honored to have been asked to be a part of *The Healing Project* and I will continue to use my voice in any way I can to fight for lung cancer awareness and the importance of its early detection. *The Healing Project* has allowed me the opportunity to once again shout the names of people who brought enormous joy into my life.

I miss my friends.

Ms. Merkerson is the star of the acclaimed TV crime drama "Law & Order." She has a long list of credits and honors including an Obie Award, a Helen Hayes Award and nominations for the Tony, Drama Desk and Image Awards.

Hope and Compassion
Lori Hope

What do you say to someone who's just been diagnosed with lung cancer? I know what people said to me:

"Oh my God! I am *so sorry*!"

And then, "Did you smoke?"

"Well, yes, I did," I would say, my eyes cast down to the floor, "but I quit seventeen years ago…" I could feel the shame burning my cheeks just as I could sense the blame clouding my questioner's compassion.

No one means to hurt someone who's been diagnosed with lung cancer. But every lung cancer survivor I've spoken with—beginning with the research for my book, *Help Me Live: 20 Things People with Cancer Want You to Know*—has told me that they have been asked that question again and again, and they have felt hurt by it, whether they smoked or not.

Why? Because when we're fighting lung cancer we're not looking back, we're looking forward. We need compassion, not blame or shame. We need support. And we need hope.

Hope is here. My name is Lori Hope. I can't take full credit for my name because I am, at least in part, Hope by design. I was born

Lori Hope Crasilneck. Funny name. People called me Spazelraz or Crazyneck when I was a kid. Well, I changed my name when I got married and then decided to change it again after my divorce. Instead of going back to Crasilneck, I decided to take on a new name. And a new identity, which I badly needed. I'd just finished making some dozen documentaries, including *Children of Cocaine*, about drug-affected babies; *Asylum in the Streets*, about the mentally ill homeless, and *Tales of Teen Parents*. Changing my name not only started some great conversations ("Are you related to Bob Hope?"); it helped me reframe the way I thought about my life.

Years later, I'm working to reframe the thinking around lung cancer. We are showing that there is hope. The recent study by Claudia Henschke, which shows an astounding 92% 10-year survival rate among people with lung cancers that are caught early and surgically removed, proves that there is great hope. We are showing that the face of cancer is not just that of an older man with a cigarette in his mouth. *Mine* is the face of lung cancer: a relatively young woman whose cancer was detected by mistake and who had a lobe of her lung cut out, before the tumor spread. We are fighting the stigma of lung cancer that has kept research on this disease woefully, shamefully underfunded.

You can help change the way we think about lung cancer. How? Let's go back to the original question: What do you say to someone who's just been diagnosed with lung cancer? Well, I doubt that we're going to stop people from asking, "Did you smoke?" But we can change the way we respond to the question. When someone asks the dreaded question, instead of politely or defensively saying, "No" or sheepishly admitting, "Yes," why not take another tack? I propose that you answer their question with a question of your own:

"Why do you ask?"

Ask the questioner to consider why she's asking and what it means. Is she worried that because she smoked or her parents smoked around her that she will get cancer? Is she attempting to blame your cancer on something you did so she will worry less about getting cancer herself? Or is the person simply affirming the very real connection between smoking and lung cancer without considering the impact the question is having on you?

I encourage you to use these questions as an opportunity to educate. To let your inquisitor know that 15 to 20 percent of lung cancers occur in people who never smoked. That 80% of those people are women. That we don't fully understand why—and that we *need* to understand.

I encourage you to take the opportunity to ask your questioner why kids in high school and college still take up smoking, and why cigarettes are still touted in movies as sophisticated or cool; why the government still subsidizes the tobacco industry and why the tobacco industry has upped the levels of nicotine in its products to ensure its victims get hooked faster and stay hooked even longer.

Use "Did you smoke?" as an opportunity. If you can. The problem is, many of us, when we have cancer and are fighting it, feel too weak and vulnerable to take a stand. We just want to go with the flow. But for those of us who can take a stand, we *must* take a stand.

How? Here's a good example. Not long ago, I was at the airport about to fly to Los Angeles to accompany my son to an appointment with an orthopedic oncologist. My son had a tumor on his leg which, the radiologist told us with 99% certainty, was not cancerous. But I was worried nonetheless. Waiting in line to board the plane, I struck up a conversation with a woman standing in front of me. She asked where I was going, and I told her about my son's condition and of our appointment in LA.

"Thank goodness they think your son's tumor is benign!" she said. "My daughter–in-law had a tumor on her leg and the leg had to be amputated." She then turned back to her husband, who had just rejoined her in line.

I felt as if a bomb had exploded inside of me. What was I to do? Write it off to another "blurt," an unintentional stab, and just let it go? I know from writing my book that one of the 20 things people with cancer most want you to know is that they need to hear success stories, not horror stories. But it's hard to communicate that directly to someone who's just told you a horror story. That's why I wrote the book, to be a voice for people touched by cancer who don't feel comfortable explaining why horror stories can cut so deep.

But this time, instead of just sucking it up, I decided to try something different. After taking a deep breath, and with compassion in my heart, I tapped the woman on her shoulder.

"I know you're a kind person," I said, "But I have to let you know that your comment terrified me, and now all I can think about is that my son's leg will have to be amputated."

"I am so sorry," she cried. "How stupid of me!"

I told her that my intention was not to make her feel awful, but to let her to know the power of her words so that she could be more careful in the future. We ended up having a great talk about it and she thanked me. We parted friends, closer for having communicated about something very difficult but very important. I was glad I had mustered up the courage to risk hurting her after she had inadvertently rocked my world.

What I learned from that experience, and what I want to share with you, is that it's okay to be assertive, and that being assertive and compassionate are not mutually exclusive. That if we can find it in ourselves to stand up for ourselves, we can help prevent others from experiencing shame, blame, terror, or trauma. And that if we can put the brakes on before telling a horror story or asking someone with lung cancer whether they smoked, we can help others and ourselves live better lives, lives of hope and compassion.

Lori Hope is an author, producer, public speaker and lung cancer survivor who quit smoking seventeen years before her diagnosis. A former newspaper editor-in-chief and award-winning journalist who developed hundreds of medical news reports and documentaries for television broadcast, her dozens of honors include two regional Emmys, a Robert F. Kennedy Journalism Award and a National Associated Press Broadcasting Award.

Lori's widely-read book, *Help Me Live: 20 Things People with Cancer Want You to Know* (Ten Speed Press/Celestial Arts, 2005), has been featured in *Redbook* magazine, *US News & World Reports*, ABC News' *Nightline* and on the Hallmark Channel, among many others. Her essays and opinion pieces have appeared in *Newsweek* and other publications and have been broadcast on hundreds of public radio stations nationwide. This essay is an adaptation of a speech given at UC San Francisco on behalf of the Lung Cancer Alliance.

Lung Cancer: What the Patient and Family Need To Know

Reed Phillips, M.D.

In 2005 there were 89,500 new lung cancer cases diagnosed in men, 74,600 in women, and 156,900 lung cancer patients succumbed to their illness. It is sad to say that, even with today's medical advances, only 14% of Americans afflicted will overcome this disease. It is small comfort that this is almost double the survival rate in Europe and the developing world, perhaps because our medical care system provides the most up to date methods of treatment. Yet we have high hopes for today's lung cancer's victims: we are on the brink of great advances in medical care for this tragic disease.

What is lung cancer? To understand the disease, we must understand how we breathe. The two lungs that form the breathing apparatus in humans consist of two parts, a branching tree of airways called *bronchi*, that brings air and oxygen to the innermost part of the lungs, and the spongy tiny cavities known as air sacs or *alveoli* which allow the transfer of oxygen to our blood, and, in return, receive carbon dioxide that is expelled from the body as a waste product.

The vast majority of lung cancers arise in either the tissue lining of these bronchi airways (*squamous cell lung cancer*) or in the glands below the surface of this lining that produce the mucus we cough up when we have a respiratory infection (*adenocarcinoma lung cancer*). With some cancers that arise in the bronchi, we are not precisely sure of the kind of cell from which the cancer originates (*large cell lung cancer*). A tiny proportion of cancers can arise from the cells forming the small air sacs themselves (*bronchioalveolar lung cancer*). Together, all of these tumors can be grouped together as *non-small cell lung cancer*, which comprise 75% of all lung cancer diagnoses. *Small cell lung cancer*, which seems to arise from nerve-like cells in the wall of the bronchial airways, makes up the remaining 25% of diagnoses. The groupings into non-small cell and small cell lung cancers are very important because the therapy used to fight the cancer and the prognosis we can expect are drastically different.

Ninety percent of all lung cancers are caused by smoking in some form. Each year, approximately 15% of the cases diagnosed in lifetime non-smokers can be attributed to exposure to second hand smoke, resulting in about 2000 deaths. This important fact indicates that many people die of lung cancer as innocent bystanders; they have done nothing to impair their own health. While there are other causes of lung cancer, all are dwarfed by smoking. The risk of contracting lung cancer for smokers is 13 times that for non-smokers (10 times the risk of the nonsmoker for a one pack per day user and 20 times the risk of the non-smoker for a 2 pack per day user).

There are no nerve endings inside the lungs. Therefore, tumor growth is often painless and undetectable. Signs of the illness can be vague and may include an unexplained cough, frequent episodes of bronchitis or multiple episodes of pneumonia, wheezing, shortness of breath, worsening of emphysema, or the spitting or coughing up of blood. A person may develop unexplained lumps in the neck, pain in the right upper abdomen above the liver area, bone or joint pains or headaches and other neurological symptoms, all of which could indicate the spread of the illness outside the chest cavity (*metastasis*). Sometimes the illness is so stealthy that the only sign might be an unexplained loss of weight, appetite, or energy.

If one develops such symptoms, he or she should immediately seek evaluation by a physician, because for the majority of the non-small cell lung cancer cases, early detection can increase the cure rate from one in seven to an encouraging 70%. Later in this book I will discuss how the patient can get the best possible care in battling his disease by acting as an educated consumer.

The history of the patient's symptoms, together with a physical exam should alert the physician to the possibility of lung cancer. The first step in diagnosis is a chest X-ray, which may or may not show the tumor. Even if the chest X-ray is negative, especially in a smoker, the doctor will order a CT scan (*Computerized Axial Tomography or computerized X-ray scan*) of the chest, a much more accurate diagnostic tool. If a tumor is seen or suspected, the physician will order appropriate blood tests or CT scans of the brain, abdomen, and sometimes pelvis to check for signs of the disease elsewhere in the body, and a bone scan, that will detect diseased areas of the skeleton. Most recently, the PET (*Positron Emission Tomography*) scan and the PET—CT scan, in which a radio-isotope is injected into the bloodstream to look for active areas of chemical metabolism that are characteristic of cancer activity, have been added to the physician's diagnostic resources.

The patient's primary physician may forgo these diagnostic tests and immediately refer the patient to a *pulmonologist*, a specialist in lung disease, who may then order these procedures. This specialist will in most cases also perform a *bronchoscopy*, where a tube of fiber optic light is inserted into the airway to locate the tumor, visualize it and obtain a piece (a *biopsy*) to determine the type of lung cancer present, which, in turn, will determine the appropriate type of therapy to be used to fight the disease. If the tumor is unreachable because it is located on the outer portions of the lungs, the physician may recommend a procedure called a *CT directed needle biopsy*, in which a radiologist, using the CT imaging machine as a guide, directs a slender needle into the tumor for a tissue sample. If it appears that the tumor is surgically removable and is still confined to the chest, the pulmonologist will use all of the available clinical findings to make a decision on whether to refer the patient to a *thoracic* (chest) *surgeon*. If the tumor is not confined to the chest, he will refer the patient to a *medical oncologist* who can treat the tumor wherever it is in the body using medications known as *chemotherapy*, or refer the patient to a *radiation oncologist* who will use high energy X-rays (*radiotherapy* or *radiation*) to attempt to eliminate or shrink the tumor.

The thoracic surgeon generally makes the decision whether the tumor can be completely excised by removing either a part of the lung or the entire lung. If the tumor has spread outside the chest, deep into the lymph nodes or into the most central portion of the bronchial network where the trachea (windpipe) divides into two branches, one to each lung, he will not operate. Nor will he operate if the tumor is found to be of the small cell type, as these tumors always spread outside the chest cavity. Even though such spread may be undetectable at the time of the tumor's diagnosis, the recurrence rate in the chest after surgery involving this form of cancer is so high that surgery is considered ineffective. The thoracic surgeon will attempt to remove the tumor if it is the more common, non-small cell cancer, if the patient is judged medically strong enough to withstand the surgery and if another procedure, the *mediastinoscopy*, done in the operating room prior to the lung operation (*thoracotomy*), confirms that the lymph glands of the central upper chest are free of any visible signs of cancer.

Chemotherapy alone cannot cure lung cancer. The only reliable way to cure lung cancer is to remove it surgically. However, if the patient is not a candidate for *resection*, or removal of the cancer, for the reasons mentioned above, or if the surgeon is unable to remove the cancer completely because it is attached to other organs and structures in the chest or involves too many lymph nodes, the patient will be sent to a medical oncologist for evaluation for chemotherapy. This physician will prescribe a selection of powerful, injectable drugs that single out the abnormal cancer cells for destruction, sometimes in combination with radiation administered by a radiation oncologist, to try to shrink the tumor. In some cases, this shrinkage is sufficient to allow the surgeon to remove the tumor. On rare occasions, radiation therapy, the use of highly energetic X-rays to destroy cancer cells, can cure a patient if the tumor is fairly localized in a small area.

If a tumor is above a certain size, the surgeon will be reluctant to remove it surgically, as the probability of its recurrence is very high due to metastases which may be present in other parts of the body. In those cases, the doctor will try to shrink the tumor with a combination of chemotherapy and radiation treatment, followed by a few months of chemotherapy only. At that point, the patient will be re-evaluated for surgical removal of the tumor. Following surgery, if the oncologist thinks there is a high risk of recurrence, she may prescribe additional rounds of chemotherapy and/or radiation.

For those patients who have symptoms that cause severe discomfort, such as bone pain, headaches, abdominal pain, difficulty in breathing, spitting up blood or shortness of breath, a course of radiation can be given for comfort and relief. All patients for whom medical technology does not allow for a cure will be offered chemotherapy to stabilize or shrink the tumor. This will afford the patient a fairly long period of comfort and good quality of life.

There is a wide variety of chemotherapy drugs, both injectable and oral and they are used in many combinations. While they are capable of causing severe side effects such as nausea, vomiting, severe fatigue, hair loss, infections, anemia and loss of appetite, other medications have been developed that reduce almost all of these symptoms, except the hair loss, so that enduring a chemotherapy regimen has been made much easier. Over the last 20 years, new forms of chemotherapy have doubled the number of lung cancer patients who live a reasonably normal life for a significant period of time and, in many cases, have tripled their life expectancy.

Unfortunately, when the tumor cannot be removed, it will eventually progress. Also, in the case of small cell lung cancers, even in the 60% to 80% of cases in which radiation and chemotherapy make the tumor disappear completely in what is known as a *complete remission*, the tumor will invariably reoccur. In these unhappy situations, the patient will have to face the final course of their illness. In the past, there was little that could be done to alleviate patients' discomfort in the last stages of lung cancer. Today, however, an entire medical science of palliative and hospice care has been developed using a wide array of medications and therapies, allowing these patients to end their days in peace. Therefore, it is essential that the medical oncologist knows when to stop the chemotherapy. Once the therapy ceases to be effective, he should work closely with the patient, the family and the palliative care and hospice specialist to make the last days of the illness peaceful and comfortable.

While today's survival rates suggest that the outlook for lung cancer patients is generally poor, we are actually on the brink of radically advanced new therapies that will be much more effective against the lung cancer cell. These will be discussed later in the book by Dr. Michael V. Smith, who will describe the amazing progress and advances that are starting to improve the outlook for patients with this disease. Furthermore, by being an educated consumer and by adopting a positive, forceful approach to this disease, the outcome can be tipped significantly in the patient's favor.

Dr. Reed Phillips is board certified in internal medicine, oncology and hospice and palliative care medicine. He is affiliated with North Shore University Hospital in New York and he is an instructor in pain management and hospice and palliative care at Winthrop University Hospital and the State University of New York School of Medicine at Stony Brook, New York.

Part II
INSPIRATION

Our lives are not determined by what happens to us but by how we react to what happens, not by what life brings to us, but by the attitude we bring to life. A positive attitude causes a chain reaction of positive thoughts, events and outcomes. It is a catalyst, a spark that creates extraordinary results.

—*Anonymous*

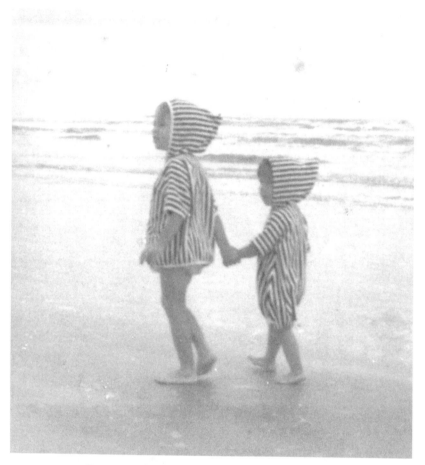

Deborah Morosini and Dana Reeve, page 29

For Dana
Deborah Morosini, M.D.

Dana Reeve, who died last winter of lung cancer, was my younger sister. I want to tell you about the terrible tragedy of her death, how it has affected her family and indeed the world, and also about the tragedy of lung cancer research and treatment today.

Dana married Superman, the actor Christopher Reeve, in 1992. She was an actor too—they met in the theatre in Williamstown, Massachusetts, where she was doing cabaret. They fell in love, married, and had a son, Will. When Will was 3, Christopher had the riding accident that resulted in his becoming paralyzed from the neck down. Dana rose to this awful crisis with the strength, grace and compassion that everyone now knows were her hallmark.

For ten years, she gave of herself fully to the care of Chris and to the CR Paralysis Foundation they established. She was tireless as a mother, too, taking their young son Will to thousands of hockey games, helping with homework, doing all of the things that mothers do, and more. All this and she was able to, a little, nurture her own career as an actor, performing in plays, television, and movies.

Chris died in October of 2004. All of us continue to grieve for this amazing man. Dana began another life as widow, caretaker of the CRP Foundation, and single mother to Will, who was then 13. She was devoted to this remarkable boy who, despite having seen his father become paralyzed, managed to grow into adolescence with strength and grace. Dana alone taught this young man not only how to survive, but to thrive in the face of tragedy.

A few months after Chris died, in the winter of 2005, our mother—Will's grandmother—passed away from cancer. She was much-loved by all. But imagine being 13 and losing your father and grandmother, who was such a huge presence in his life, in the space of only 4 months. Imagine being Dana, who was only 42, losing her beloved husband, and her own mother, in such a short time.

And then imagine, the following summer, when you feel that life just might begin to turn around ... that you just might be able to begin again ... you're feeling youthful, beautiful, maybe, finally, even a little happy ... you see your son growing into a man and you're feeling that he's growing up just right ... you're still in mourning for your husband and mother, naturally, but it's summer, and the future seems bright with possibilities ... you're feeling these things, but you also have a little cough that won't go away. As if something's stuck in your throat. You think it's nothing, but it's annoying. And you tell your doctor about it, and he checks it out, and you discover that you have lung cancer.

And you tell your son about it.

And you tell your sisters and your father about it.

And seven months later... you're gone.

We are a family of physicians. My father is a doctor, his father was a doctor and I am a doctor. In medical school, I learned a bit about lung cancer—how complicated it is, how many different versions of it exist, how difficult it is to treat. I learned how high the mortality rate is for lung cancer. When I found out that Dana had it—well, I hardly have words to express how devastated I was ... for myself, for all the people in the world who so loved her, but mostly for her son, Will, rendered fatherless and motherless within the space of less than two years. Can you imagine?

There is tremendous ignorance about the facts of lung cancer and about its treatment. Even I, as a physician who works in research every day, was unaware of the facts until I had to face Dana's tragedy.

Lung cancer is the single biggest cancer killer worldwide. It accounts for one third of all cancer deaths in this country. One third. I'll say it again: one third. This is more than all other cancer deaths combined—breast, prostate, colon, kidney, melanoma. Lung cancer takes more lives than any other cancer.

And yet lung cancer research receives the least amount of federal funding of any cancer. For example, although lung cancer accounts for twice as many deaths among women as breast cancer, breast cancer research receives 13 times as much federal funding. This, despite the fact that 70% of the patients diagnosed with lung cancer will not survive more than a few months and only 15% will live for five more years or longer.

There is no question that most lung cancer cases are smoking-related. But my sister was one of the 15% or so of all victims who *never* smoked. Fifty percent of all lung cancer cases are of former smokers—people who may have given up smoking years ago. And the rest are current smokers.

Is it right that lung cancer research funding is so paltry because of the stigma we associate with smoking? Remember, about 60% of all new cases are of people who had never smoked, or who had given up smoking years before. Is the lack of funding due to an attitude that lung cancer patients somehow deserve the disease, because they were smokers? If so, we need to change this perception.

As the proud sister of Dana Reeve, it is my way of honoring her and all of those affected by lung cancer to now make this my life's work: to raise a loud voice for lung cancer research and support and to carry on her legacy of strength and compassion. In my work as a research physician, and now as a spokeswoman for lung cancer victims, I owe Dana, and you, this future. It is most surely what she would have wanted.

———————————

Doctor Morosini is a pathologist working in the field of translational medicine, a branch of medical research focused on "translating" basic research findings into real therapies for real patients. A graduate of Boston University School of Medicine, Dr. Morosini is a spokesperson for and a member of Lung Cancer Alliance. She lives with her family in the Boston area.

It All Depends
on Your Attitude
Ed Levitt

Two years ago I was diagnosed with Stage IV lung cancer. Before then, I enjoyed a full and productive life. My wife and I were making plans for our retirement. It was very important to us because, as some would say, I was a workaholic. I felt ready to make a change and start doing the things for which we had waited so long.

I had a wonderful career as an international speaker and motivator. I spoke to major corporations and groups of five to five thousand people. It was an exciting and demanding life. I never wanted to stop. To be honest, I didn't think I could stop. I always worked hard and never found time to play. I promised my wife we were going to make up for lost time when I retired. We thought of moving back to Chattanooga, a place we both loved. Unfortunately, events altered our great plans: the stock market crashed at the most inopportune time and my retirement was put on hold until I reached sixty-five.

Initially, this was devastating. But it was only money, not our health or our lives, so I planned to work as long as I could. I was not going to let this get me down. We tried to comfort ourselves by remembering that both our families are long-lived. My father died at ninety and my mother had just passed away at one hundred. I had taken only four or five sick days off of work in over thirty years. I never even took an aspirin. I just didn't get sick.

I did smoke for a few years, but that was 34 years ago. I didn't think smoking was a problem because there is no cancer in my family and everybody smoked in the 1950's and 60's. Even my doctors offered his patients a cigarette to relax. Back then, every hospital room had ashtrays.

I focused on exercise to make sure I would be in outstanding physical condition when I retired. I did aerobics, kickboxing, spinning, weights, some yoga and walked daily. I was in outstanding shape. I believed that when illness strikes, you must be in good condition to fight back. I believed the old adage, "A strong mind and body are the keys for survival."

But in spite of all the things I did right, just as I was ready to retire and enjoy life, I found out that I had lung cancer. The last week in January, 2003, I was getting off a plane in Las Vegas to attend a convention. Walking from the plane to baggage claim, I developed a severe pain in the groin area of my right leg. Because I exercised so much, I was used to aches and pains, so I ignored it. However, as the days went on, the pain grew worse and I started to limp. Towards the end of the convention I was spending forty minutes sitting on the floor of my hotel bathroom just to put my pants on.

When I returned home, my wife insisted that I go to a doctor. We decided on a young graduate doctor because we thought she would be thorough, and she was. Because of my active lifestyle, she thought I had some inflammation due to over-exertion, and she prescribed anti-inflammatory medication. She told me that if there was no change in two weeks, she would want to see me again.

One week later, I revisited the doctor with a hard lump in the right side of my groin. She immediately ordered a chest X-ray, blood tests, a CT scan, MRI, a bone scan and sent me to an oncology surgeon for a biopsy. The X-ray showed a spot, so they did it again. The bone scan showed tumors on my spine, ribs, neck, and collar bone. The CT scan showed lung spots and large tumors on both adrenal glands.

The cancer was moving fast. By then, I had developed severe pain everywhere. My face was drooping so severely on one side that a specialist said I had palsy. I had unbearable neck and back pain. I did not know how to get comfortable. I consulted with a supposedly very good oncologist. He read the test results and called us into his office. He walked in, gave me a very cold look and said, "You have Stage IV lung cancer, it's terminal, there is nothing we can do for you. Get your affairs in order and make funeral arrangements. You have about 60 to 90 days." His beeper went off. He looked up and said, "I must leave now, I have to be at my son's school or my wife will be furious. Any questions, call me or come in tomorrow." He left. I was given a 90-day death sentence and my doctor had to be at his son's school. How was I supposed to feel? I had never cried in my life, but I did then. I was scared and didn't know what to do. I was lost.

People kept telling me they knew how I felt. How could they possibly know? Best friends began to stay at arm's length. I heard things like, "Please don't breathe on me, I don't want cancer," or "It's your own fault because you smoked."

My wife refused to take this lying down. She immediately made an appointment for a second opinion. I met the doctor. After he reviewed all of my charts, I said, "Doc, is there even a little hope, anything?" He looked back at me with a cold, waxy look and the enthusiasm of a one-eyed mortician and said, "There is always hope."

I had to make a decision. I had to decide if I would lie down and let it take over what life I had left or stand up and fight it on my terms. No one can do it for you, since no one knows what you are going through. Maybe we won't live as long as we originally expected, maybe we will. We don't know. At that moment I knew

I was at a crossroads and I chose life. I decided to help the doctors help all other lung cancer patients in the future. I wanted to leave a legacy. It was important to me that I try and make a difference. I would not sit around feeling sorry for myself.

My life has changed in ways that I could never have imagined. Retirement in the normal sense will never come. I can't work because nobody wants a sick man who must go to the hospital regularly or is bald because of the big "C." In our society, cancer makes you a leper. Everybody wants to tell you about somebody they know who died of lung cancer or how they are suffering with lung cancer. Strangers call just to tell you about a lung cancer death. "Did you hear about Peter Jennings?" Everybody admires you, from a distance. "More than ninety days, and you're still around, wow!"

The doctors told me it was because I was in such good shape that I was able to fight the disease. They told me if I kept moving it would help me stay alive. As hard as it was, I started walking an hour at a time. The chemotherapy I was receiving made me very weak and tired, and as I walked I would hold onto mailboxes and throw up. I fell down many times, but I got up again and again, and I kept walking. I increased my walks to about three hours every day. I then added water aerobics at the YMCA. I was the only man among all of the "blue haired ladies" in the pool. But I was getting stronger.

After three months of chemotherapy, a CT scan showed that my cancer had spread. I thought my life was over. But then I began radiation and started on the drug Iressa. Three months later, I had another scan and this time my cancer was reduced by 70%. The two large tumors in my adrenal glands were gone. My face was back to normal (my family may dispute the word "normal" when I talk about my face!)

My hospital started a lung cancer support group and I attended. I was at my wit's end after a few meetings: all we talked about was our disease and how we felt. It was my monthly Doom and

Gloom. Finally, at a meeting that August I stood up and said, "No more. I need to give back. I need to help the researchers at my hospital because the researchers are helping me. If I am going to take, then I am going to give back."

I jumped in with both feet. I offered my speaking skills to any group that would listen. I asked my hospital what I could do to help. I joined the Lung Cancer Alliance in Washington, D.C., the only group that is solely focused on lung cancer advocacy. I became the lead LCA advocate in the State of Georgia and, at the time I write this, I am forming the Lung Cancer Alliance— Georgia, a group that is tied in with all hospitals and oncologists in the state. We are here to make a difference. I am working with my hospital to aggressively pursue research dollars and raise awareness of lung cancer. I am meeting with congressmen, senators, and state representatives. We are working directly with pharmaceutical companies and speaking in support of lung cancer research. We are coordinating all hospitals and oncologists to join in our fight. We are scheduled to have our first annual celebrity golf tournament and a black tie dinner and dance to raise funds. What about license plates for lung cancer? It can be done. The list goes on and on. My life is devoted to helping to find a cure, or if not, then at least developing medication that can control lung cancer, a method for early detection and to increase funding for research.

My aggressive business nature is still focused to win, but now it is to beat cancer. As you can imagine, time is not something I take for granted. I am more active and feel better now than I have in years. Because I don't take it for granted, I can now have quality of life and I can have it as long as I keep fighting. I hear things I never heard before when walking my greyhounds. I see things very differently. I see the "true" color of flowers. I feel from my heart. Oh, I still have Stage IV lung cancer, but between my hospital and my medication, I have been given time. How much time, nobody knows.

Do I hurt? Do I have bad days? Yes. But it is not about me. It is about staying alive to help beat lung cancer, to help the millions who will follow me with this disease. When speaking to groups or individuals I tell them that the medication is only 50% and attitude and exercise are the other 50%. If I do not fight, who will? For some reason, most lung cancer patients are not fighters, but just accept their fate. I encourage them to fight on their terms to win. Projects like this book will make a huge difference. I am proud to help even one person to fight and stay alive, if not longer, then at least with quality of life, with dignity.

Born in London during the Second World War, Ed is a professional motivational speaker who resides in the Greater Atlanta area.

Editor's Note: In the months since his diagnosis, the author founded the Lung Cancer Alliance-GA to promote awareness at both the state and national level. He partnered with his hospital's Lung Cancer Oncology research group to raise funds for research. He has been a keynote speaker for the Emory-Winship Cancer Center, and a story highlighting his efforts was recently published in Emory's semi-annual magazine *Winship-Report.* He was the subject of a full page story in the *Atlanta Journal Constitution.* He appeared on *CNN* when Dana Reeve died of lung cancer.

Ed was instrumental in the enactment of a Senate resolution declaring lung cancer a national public health priority. He is currently working with Georgia state senators to pass legislation to include lung cancer on state income tax forms as an optional donation. He is working with Georgia legislators to create a state license plate for lung cancer, with proceeds going to lung cancer research. He has worked with the Lung Cancer Alliance National to reinstate Iressa as a first-line targeted therapy for patients with lung cancer and he helped secure a resolution, passed in the Georgia senate, making November "Lung Cancer Awareness Month."

A Patient's Mission
Jennifer Daly
Nicholyn Hutchinson

Tammy Willett had always been the "pied piper" among her family and friends in her insistence on prevention and early detection of breast cancer. She even earned the nickname "the mammogram police," because whenever Tammy would make her annual appointment for a mammogram, she would also schedule appointments for her sister and friends. She was equally attentive to skin cancer prevention and early detection. "I'd get my moles checked every year," she recalls. In addition to having regular check-ups and screenings, she lived a healthy lifestyle and was a non-smoker. Her vigilance gave her a sense of security, believing that she was doing everything possible to ensure that she was cancer-free. Having taken every precaution, Tammy could not imagine the event that would come to change her life forever.

Upon returning from an overseas trip in March 2005, Tammy developed shortness of breath. "I was in Miami at the time. I could hardly breathe. I thought I had bronchitis," she remembers. Still experiencing symptoms when she arrived back in Georgia, she stopped by a local drop-in clinic near her office. The clinic's doctor suggested a lung X-ray, but unfortunately Tammy's insurance would not cover it. Still not feeling well, she decided to pay for the X-ray herself. "I expected to get an antibiotic and go about my business," she says. Instead, her X-ray revealed a significant amount of fluid in her lung. She was immediately taken by ambulance to the intensive care unit of a nearby hospital. Tammy had never before been admitted to a hospital other than for her daughter's birth.

On March 15, Tammy was diagnosed with Stage III lung cancer. On March 22, she traveled out of state to a renowned cancer center. Once the physicians there learned where she lived, they advised her to go home to Georgia, telling her that some of the best doctors specializing in lung cancer were right in her own backyard: medical oncologists Michael Fanucchi, MD, and Fadlo Khuri, MD, both at Winship Cancer Institute of Emory University in Atlanta. Knowing time was of the essence, the next day she drove straight from the airport to Winship.

Six rounds of chemotherapy later, Willett's cancer was termed "inactive." Given her history of good health, her diagnosis begs the question: why does a healthy non-smoker get lung cancer? Tammy doesn't know, nor do her doctors. However, for her, the "why" is not her focus—living is. Living strong after her diagnosis, Tammy is now focused on raising money for lung cancer research. A few months ago, she teamed up with Ed Levitt, another lung cancer survivor she met through Winship's Lung Cancer Support Group. Now, more than 18 months after his own diagnosis of Stage IV lung cancer, Levitt has become a tireless advocate for raising funds for lung cancer research.

In their determination and courage to fight and not give up, Tammy and Ed are surviving a disease that kills more people than colon, breast, and prostate cancers combined. Lung cancer is the leading cause of cancer death among both men and women in the state of Georgia and in the United States. Yet, despite these daunting facts, lung cancer currently receives the smallest amount of research funding of all major cancers. A formidable and passionate duo, Tammy and Ed have dedicated their lives to changing this fact. This past October, they were instrumental in having Georgia Governor Sonny Purdue officially designate November Lung Cancer Awareness Month in the state.

In addition to her lung cancer advocacy, Tammy's life is centered around Bailey, her nine-year-old daughter, her passionate love for travel, providing support to her husband John's business and her job of more than eighteen years with an Atlanta area land development company. Together with her daughter and husband, she has a wonderful support system in her sister Kathy and close friend Elaina, both of whom have accompanied her to every doctor's appointment.

A doting mother, Tammy attends every one of her daughter's softball games and horse riding competitions. For Columbus Day weekend, they traveled to New York. Avid Braves fans, they went to the playoff game in Atlanta despite a tropical storm drenching the city prior to the game. Most recently, Tammy planned the Halloween party of all Halloween parties for 40 of her daughter's friends and their parents. In August 2006, she took a trip to Africa with her husband, daughter, sister and niece. She spreads hope and joy wherever she goes and the energy with which she lives life rivals the energy of most people who have never been diagnosed with cancer.

"Through all this, with the exception of the chemo, I haven't felt bad" she says. As her battle with lung cancer continues, she is the picture of strength. In fact, when you experience Tammy's tireless energy and positive outlook, it's easy not to think about what she has faced this past year, even as her battle continues.

Addressing her newfound purpose in life, raising funding levels and awareness for lung cancer research, Tammy says, "when something like this happens, sometimes you can find yourself wondering 'Why me?' But maybe this is why. Maybe I am supposed to bring attention to this terrible disease. I know this is my mission now."

Jennifer Daly is the Director of Major Gifts for Emory University's Winship Cancer Institute in Atlanta, GA. A graduate of the University of Georgia's Grady College of Journalism and Mass Communication, Ms. Daly has worked in higher education for more than 15 years through work in public relations, research communications, international relations, and development.

Nicholyn Hutchinson is Senior Editor at Emory University's Winship Cancer Institute. Her writing career began when she won, at age 8, her elementary school poetry contest. With two graduate degrees in English from the University of Georgia, she has published both fiction and non-fiction works and is currently at work on a children's book.

God Doesn't Pull You Through a Jam So You Can Keep It For Yourself

Lea Sopkin

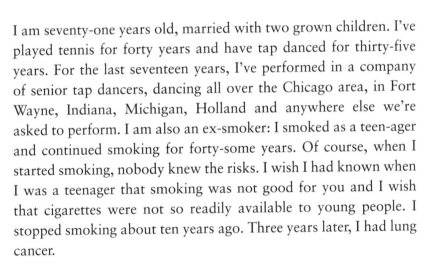

I am seventy-one years old, married with two grown children. I've played tennis for forty years and have tap danced for thirty-five years. For the last seventeen years, I've performed in a company of senior tap dancers, dancing all over the Chicago area, in Fort Wayne, Indiana, Michigan, Holland and anywhere else we're asked to perform. I am also an ex-smoker: I smoked as a teen-ager and continued smoking for forty-some years. Of course, when I started smoking, nobody knew the risks. I wish I had known when I was a teenager that smoking was not good for you and I wish that cigarettes were not so readily available to young people. I stopped smoking about ten years ago. Three years later, I had lung cancer.

I had what I described to my doctor as a "killer cough." I'd had this kind of cough many times in the past, but for some reason, this time my doctor told me to get a chest X-ray. The results were inconclusive, so she set up a CT scan. The results indicated a malignant tumor on one kidney and an anomaly in the left lung. A biopsy revealed a malignant tumor on the lung and confirmed the tumor found on my kidney. I underwent every possible scan and test to determine whether both cancers were primary or had spread from one to the other and if the cancer had spread elsewhere in my body. At the end of all this testing, the two cancers were, indeed, determined to be primary, but had not spread anywhere else, caught in the very early stages. My oncologist told me, "The bad news is that we have to remove one kidney and a lobe of one lung, but the good news is that no other treatment will be necessary because the cancers are contained." So, seven years ago, I had the two surgeries one month apart and I have been cancer-free ever since.

I survived because of very early detection by my two guardian angels: my primary doctor, who responded to her gut feeling and quickly sent me for tests, and the radiologist who read the CT scan for my lung and found the cancer on my kidney. Without them, I don't know if I would be here today. I am grateful to all the people I know who prayed for me in all their different religions and for the love and support of my family and friends, especially my husband and daughter, who were there for me and with me every step of the way.

My prognosis for the moment is good. However, I get CT scans every year and I keep my fingers crossed until I get the results. I guess you never really feel as though you're out of the woods after going through this.

People need to know about early detection, when lung cancer is most curable. I would advise anyone diagnosed with lung cancer to get whatever help they can and to have a positive attitude. I had a positive attitude, and it helped me get though this ordeal.

The author is a 73-year-old mother of two who has played tennis and tap danced for 40 years. For the last 19 years she has been a member of a company of senior tap dancers, performing in Illinois, Indiana and Michigan.

Elisabeth

Misha Segal

> "Everything happens for a reason and even if sometimes things
> seem to make no sense, the future reveals why it happened."
>
> —*Elisabeth Buchhalter Segal*

I grew up listening to those words by my mother Elisabeth; my
mother, who was also my best friend and inspiration to my work
as a composer.

Elisabeth was born in Vienna on October 31, 1920. (Many years
later she would learn that day was celebrated far away by an
entire country dressed up in funny costumes. She was tickled!) As
a teenager, Elisabeth was Austria's table tennis champion. At the
age of 17 she played against one of Germany's toughest competi-
tors. Elisabeth won the first set, at which point her opponent
threw her racket at the table, uttering, "I will not play against a
filthy Jew." Thanks to the anti-Semitic propaganda machine, all
Jews had been degraded into an unclean caricature of hooked
noses and large lips. A gasp could be heard from the audience at
the opponent's revelation: it was hard for everybody, including the
judges, to believe that this young Austrian blond beauty, who
looked to them more like Rita Hayworth's sister than the propa-

ganda they were so familiar with, was really a Jew. Elisabeth's membership to the sports club was revoked there and then.

In 1938, Hitler invaded Austria. Elisabeth witnessed beatings on the street, men dragged by their beards for all to see. Her own skin melted off her fingers from being forced to scrub the streets and Nazi army barracks with lye and acid. Her parents, prominent business and property owners, refused to leave but urged their daughters to run. Grete, their oldest, made it to Australia. Elisabeth's first attempt to escape was thwarted. Her second attempt at the end of 1938 was successful, but very difficult: she and several hundred others traveled for more than two months on three different small, dirty boats manned by pirates who helped themselves to jewelry, shoes, whatever they could get their hands on. Final destination: The Promised Land. The last boat anchored about 10 kilometers from the shores of Nathanya. It could not get close to the shore because British soldiers were guarding the beach; they were known for sending Jews—who were attempting to "illegally" enter the land—back to Europe, back to the camps. But Jews already inhabiting the land tricked the Brits with booze and women, creating a distraction just long enough so all could jump ship and swim to freedom. It took several hours to account for everyone but they all made it.

That was my mother.

Elisabeth lost her parents to the Nazis but found strength to start a new life in Israel, where she met my Russian father and where I was born. She learned to laugh and live again. Her spirit could not be broken. In fact, after the war she was sent to Austria as part of a ping-pong team to represent the newly born state of Israel, the only girl amongst 11 men. She beat the Austrian champion in an exhibition game. Being just a few years after the war, the audience was still full of Nazis. The Israeli team wore the blue and white flag of their country, the Star of David, on their shirts and jackets. Elisabeth writes in her memoir, "…the same symbol they called

'Judenstern' which we had to wear as a sign of degradation and an invitation for anyone to abuse and torture us. Now we brought honor and respect to our beloved symbol and our flag."

That was my mother's spirit.

Elisabeth went on to lead a wonderful, rich life, traveling around the world, learning 5 different languages, doing international business and settling in New York City. It was many years later, in 1995, that Elisabeth was diagnosed with lung cancer. She had been coughing for a year. Her doctor insisted she had a pulmonary infection and so kept her on antibiotics for several months. When her condition did not improve, she insisted upon an X-ray. That's when the tumor was discovered. It was big and delicately placed. She came to Los Angeles to have an operation to remove the affected lung. The operation was fruitless: the cancer had already spread to the lining of the chest and removing it would not solve the problem.

Her first oncologist gave her 6 months to live. As soon as he uttered the words "You should start preparing..." Elisabeth got up and walked right out. "Where are you going, Mama?" I asked. "*He* can start preparing" she said, "*I* am not going anywhere, definitely not in six months!"

We found another oncologist at USC/Norris, Dr. Isaiah Dimery, who was more encouraging. Elisabeth stayed around for six years, almost an unheard of victory, considering that the disease was quite advanced. Dr. Dimery became one of Elisabeth's best friends and remains my personal friend to this day. "She is one of a kind," he used to say. "If I had a bad day, Elisabeth would force a smile on my face. She would give *me* encouragement when it was *she* who actually needed it the most."

That was my Mama.

How did she do it? Straight from the hospital, on the way home, a day after open lung surgery, Elisabeth asked me, "Aren't we stopping for coffee?" She never let her physical condition interfere with her life. She never complained. As a matter of fact, after a chemotherapy session, Elisabeth would "spite" the cancer and go to a Broadway show or a concert of the New York Philharmonic. I would come for visits in New York and she would out-walk me. "Shouldn't we sit down a second?" I would ask after a 35-block walk on the Upper West Side. She'd look at me as if I'd just suggested the unthinkable. "Mishinka, if we sit down, we're going to be late for the movies...."

Over the years, we visited each other often and quite frankly, she was taking this much better than I was! I did everything I could for her; researched the latest treatments and clinical trials; accompanied her to important doctor visits and of course, played piano for her (if you are familiar with my *Female* CDs, that is the music I played for her), but it was she who kept the light shining long after the darkness came in.

That was Mama.

In the last year, Elisabeth was forced to slow down so I asked her to move in with me, my wife and our baby. Kicking and screaming, she left the city she loved. Upon arrival in Los Angeles, Mama, of course, continued to take care of me, ordering my (now ex) wife around if she fell short of her standards for how the house should be held; staying up with my friends and me until 2 a.m., drinking wine, talking politics and art.

It was only in the last 3 months that she became everything I didn't recognize my mother to be. Yet, her eyes still shone and painful as it was, her smile could still light up a room.

One night in the last week before she departed, she was feeling especially sick. She asked to see her oncologist, Dr. Ronald Natale from Cedars-Sinai, so I called him. He came to the house, checked her and told me this was the end of the road. When I called the next day to thank him for coming by, his assistant was dumbfounded: "Dr. Natale went to your home to see Elisabeth?" she asked. "Yes" was my answer, "and I wanted to thank him, it meant a lot to her". "I'll be darned," she said, "I have been working for him for over ten years and he's never, ever made a house call." Later I asked Dr. Natale about that. His reply was, "I have never had a patient like Elisabeth before. I would come into the room and she would insist on finding out how *I* was doing. She never complained, was never phased by her condition. I came because I knew that if Elisabeth needed to see me, she must have really been in bad shape, so I *had* to see her."

Mother's Day, 2001 marked the day Elisabeth Buchhalter Segal left our lives.

The next year, to honor what would have been her 82nd birthday, I played a concert at Cedars-Sinai for the cancer patients. Dr. Natale saw Elisabeth's picture on the piano and his eyes welled. That concert was the first of many around the country and none of them would have happened if it weren't for Elisabeth. Even after her departure, she's giving, giving, giving to other people. Elisabeth did not "fight" the disease. Her victory lies within the fact that she wouldn't grant it any importance. "My life comes first. Diseases—they come last on my priority list."

Elisabeth Buchhalter Segal was my mother, my best friend, forever my inspiration…and maybe yours, now, too.

After studying film, philosophy and music at Tel Aviv University, Misha apprenticed under 20th century master composer Dieter Schöhnbach in Germany, studied composition and conducting at the Guildhall School of Music in London and graduated from the Berklee College of Music. In his native Israel, Misha's jazz, rock and pop influences helped change the face of popular music, garnering numerous #1 hits. His classical compositions have been performed by the Israeli Philharmonic and the Israel Chamber Ensemble. Misha has created, composed and conducted scores for a variety of feature films including *The Phantom of the Opera*, and the all time favorite kids' movie, *The New Adventures of Pippi Longstocking*. Also to his credit are numerous works for the small screen, which earned him an Emmy® Award.

His solo piano collection, *Red, White & Blue Female* is the core of Misha's *Beauty Found in Unlikely Places* concert series. The concerts and the music were inspired by his mother, a woman with an unbreakable spirit. Through these concerts, associated media interviews and Public Service Announcements, he forwards his mission of educating the public on lung cancer awareness issues and raising the quality of life of those fighting the biggest battle of theirs.

Joan's Story
Patrick McNeive

Joan Scarangello discovered a whole new world when she was diagnosed with lung cancer in 2000 at the age of 46.

A serious, driven broadcast news writer, she freed herself from the bonds of work, and became able, for the first time in her life; to do the things she wanted to do when she wanted to do them. She lunched with old friends, worked on her novel, relaxed in her summer cottage, got married and all the while she focused on keeping herself as healthy as possible. She was active until the week she died. Unhampered by chemotherapy, relapses, hair and weight loss, she was determined to make the best of the time she had left.

Joan had just nine months from the time of her diagnosis with Stage IV lung cancer until her death. But many of her closest friends agree that she had never had a happier time, or a period when she'd been so at peace with the world. Joan had seen lung cancer 20 years earlier, when she watched her mother (another non-smoker) die of the disease after a short, brave fight. Yet she was not remotely affected by fear of the disease. Rather, she was energized by the power of life and love and the possibilities for joy that each waking minute could bring.

Early in her diagnosis, Joan was fortunate to meet Barbara Parisi, a firebrand of a woman and an open advocate for lung cancer victims. Barbara was the "poster child" for lung cancer victims, having survived more than a year and, as it turned out, more than five years until her death in 2004. Barbara's success gave Joan hope. Her passion to fight the disease inspired Joan's strength and her compassion gave Joan comfort. Together, they became warriors to fight for a cure—for themselves and others.

Joan never let lung cancer get in the way of her top priority: family. During a visit to the emergency room at Memorial Sloan Kettering, she hurried the nurses along so that she would not be late for Thanksgiving dinner with them. She traveled to California during her illness to attend the christening of her godchild and to spend more time with her West Coast relatives. She insisted always on including her stepdaughter, Franny, in every phase of her life. She planned our wedding down to the last detail, to make it a celebration that would embody her hopefulness and belief in love everlasting. We were all caught up in the dream of that day, feeling, perhaps, in those hours the way Joan did throughout her illness.

Joan did not finish her novel, but her writing put her life in focus and strengthened her will to beat the odds. She surrounded her desk with inspirational writings. The one that struck me the most and which she had taped onto her laptop was: "Your soul will be attended to by your very lucky family and friends."

We did not have enough time with Joan. But her too-short life will have a long-term impact—not just on those of us who knew her, but also on the landscape of lung cancer research, treatment and the search for a cure. In her honor and memory, and to keep our promise to help her fight the disease, we created *Joan's Legacy: the Joan Scarangello Foundation to Conquer Lung Cancer*. In just five years, Joan's Legacy has become a leading resource in the search for new treatments and a cure for lung cancer and the end to the smoking-related stigma that plagues victims of the lung cancer diagnosis. The first nonprofit in the U.S. to identify and cultivate lung cancer research, with a special focus on raising awareness of non-tobacco-related lung cancer, Joan's Legacy has quickly become recognized as the "venture capital" for lung cancer research in the U.S. We will have awarded more than $2 million in research grants by the end of 2006.

A cure for lung cancer will be found. And it will be Joan's Legacy.

Patrick McNeive is the husband of Joan Scarangello and the President of Joan's Legacy: the Joan Scarangello Foundation to Conquer Lung Cancer.

Taking Charge of Your Care

Reed Phillips, MD

You are a patient and you have been told that the cause of your shortness of breath, spitting of blood, unexplained weight loss or the shadow on your chest X-ray has been found. Your physician schedules an appointment with you to explain the results of the tests. You are hoping for the best but you suspect the news will not be good: most patients whose symptoms require a complex set of medical tests to enable a diagnosis are already thinking and worrying about cancer. Your mind is churning with possibilities. What will the doctor say? How bad is it? Will I die? Are there any treatments available? What will this mean to my family? Your mind is racing with anxiety and fear.

My purpose in writing this essay is to explain to the medical consumer, be it the patient or the patient's advocate or caregiver, how to negotiate the healthcare system, manage the patient's care and maximize the chances of overcoming this disease. The key is to take control, and not let the system control you. The healthcare system is a very complex, intimidating maze of physicians, laboratory tests, facilities, forms, insurance companies and regulations which, to the uninitiated, may present serious obstacles to receiving the best care for and management of the disease. Many simply lack the information to effectively navigate the system. Equally important, no one has told them about the importance of the positive, "kick-ass" attitude needed to beat this illness.

Continued on page (72)

Life is Great,
One Day at a Time

Dave Grant

I was in the United States Army during the Vietnam War. I worked with a team that handled the transport of blood supplies to wounded soldiers. Although this was a stressful and often heart wrenching job, I put my entire self into it. I was helping, in the only way I could at that time, men and women who were fighting for our country.

Looking back now, I realize that although this was an extremely difficult time for me, it led to one of my life's greatest blessings. My wife, an Army Personnel Specialist, was working right along with me. From the beginning of our relationship we shared both the worst of times and what soon became the best of times. During our time in Vietnam together, we learned the acceptance and coping skills that have bonded us through thick and thin for the last thirty-five years. Our marriage has been blessed with two lovely children.

I mention the distant past because it plays such a vital role in the life I have lived for the last few years. I didn't know that in later years, the things I witnessed back then would help me appreciate my life even more today. Many times in recent years when I was feeling down, memories of those young soldiers with arms missing or legs amputated made me feel blessed, even in the midst of my own chronic illness.

Five years ago this fall, the results of a needle biopsy confirmed that I had lung cancer. On October 8, 2001, I had surgery to remove the lower and upper lobes of my right lung. At a follow-up appointment in July 2002, another tumor was found in the same general area as the first. I had a consultation with both my thoracic surgeon and my oncologist, and we decided to go back in and see what was going on. In the second surgery they found benign tumors, which, I was told, may have been due to scarring from the first surgery.

Shortly afterwards I went to the University of Wisconsin Comprehensive Cancer Center for a second opinion with Dr. Joan Schiller, founder of the National Lung Cancer Partnership. At the conclusion of the appointment I asked if I could continue with her as my primary oncologist. She agreed and a great relationship has followed. I know now that although no doctors have all the answers, finding the right one for you makes all the difference.

In April 2003, at a surgery follow-up appointment, I was told that the cancer had metastasized throughout much of my lymphatic system. A biopsy of two lymph nodes in my neck revealed that it was from the lung cancer. I was immediately started on various drugs. A CT scan at the end of September revealed that the tumors had either disappeared or had stabilized. However, a few months later, a CT scan revealed a tumor in my liver.

I entered a trial with a new drug. It was a double blind study, so at first I didn't know which drug I was getting. After about six weeks on the study drug, I developed side effects and was removed from the trial. The good part was that in January 2004, a CT scan revealed that the liver tumor was stable. I was scanned monthly throughout the remainder of 2004, and it remained stable.

The following January, I received bad news. A new tumor was growing in the lower lobe of my right lung. The decision was made to follow the growth of the tumor with monthly scans. By March 30, 2005, the tumor had doubled in size to approximately two centimeters. On June 8, 2005 I entered a Phase I trial for Sutent, a new drug. I have continued to take the drug in cycles, fourteen days on the drug and seven days off. This will continue for an indefinite period of time. The good news is that I am now stable.

For sure, my life has been like a roller coaster. There were times when I'd get bad medical news and I'd feel like the bottom was falling out of my world. Then I'd receive news that a tumor had shrunk or that I had stabilized, and I would mentally fly way up high. Being human, at first I voiced the expected, "Why me?" I no longer wonder why. My experiences with lung cancer have enabled me to help others around me who have had to deal with the disease. I have been active on the Internet as well, having joined several lung cancer message boards. I look forward to finding new friends and continuing with many old friends from other web sites.

I really believe that the one thing necessary to beat lung cancer is to educate doctors. We need to make them aware of new treatments that are out there. I try to do my part by communicating with others in chat rooms, by sending e-mails, or posting on bulletin boards.

While the ride on life's roller coaster has indeed been scary, I thank God every day that He didn't expect me to go it alone. Every time I had good test results, my best friend, my wife, made the ride to the top with me. Invariably, each time I started hurtling downward, she would somehow beat me to the bottom and be there waiting for me. We have learned the importance of laughing and crying together. When I speak at group meetings I always like to stress that spouses of people with any illness need support too.

I credit my being alive and active today to my beautiful family and friends who have supported me in ways I can't even begin to write about. My religion and spirituality are extremely important to me and I truly believe that a positive attitude can make all the difference in the world. My life, even with lung cancer, has been truly great. In a sense, I believe I have had the best of the best. I wake up each morning and thank God for giving me yet one more day. I am still alive, I have my wife and two children and together we will make life better in our corner of the world.

_____

The writer retired from the United States Army as Sergeant First Class. He celebrated five years of cancer survivorship on September 11, 2006 and is State Representative for Wisconsin in the Lung Cancer Alliance.

My Story

Debra Violette

In April 1998, I came down with a cold. By the end of the weekend I was coughing up specks of blood. I called my doctor, who prescribed antibiotics and scheduled an appointment with me for the following Thursday to see how I was doing. When we met, I told him I was still coughing up blood and not feeling as well as I should after being on antibiotics. He sent me to the hospital for an X-ray and told me to wait there until it had been read. He called me at the hospital after the radiologist read the film to tell me that there was something on my right lower lobe. He scheduled a CT scan for the next day and an appointment with a pulmonary specialist on Monday.

The pulmonary specialist asked me a battery of questions. He led me down a hall to his office, where he placed the film on the light box. He turned around and said, "This is the first time I have seen these. You have lung cancer." When I heard that, I thought, no one survives lung cancer. I am going to die.

Because of the stigma attached to this disease, I was very reluctant to discuss my sickness. I was afraid of what people would say or think. I finally got up the nerve to tell my family, friends, and supervisor. I was overwhelmed by the support I got from colleagues, friends and people whom I did not even know. Family members were not as supportive: they were experiencing their own issues surrounding my diagnosis and could not give me the support I needed.

I was referred to the Dana-Farber Cancer Institute in Boston for further testing and staging. It was finally determined that I had Stage III-A non-small-cell lung cancer. This is a rather late stage diagnosis with a 10% chance of survival past five years. They told me I would need three rounds of chemotherapy, and my right lower lobe removed if the tumors responded to chemo and 25 rounds of radiation.

I went back to Maine and started my first round of chemotherapy in June. I was terribly ill the second day after treatment, and felt as if someone had beaten my entire body with a baseball bat. I did not see how I could go through two more rounds of chemotherapy feeling like this, but the symptoms went away almost as suddenly as they had come on.

In July, I had my second round of chemotherapy. I began to lose my hair. This was a very emotional part of my treatment; however, I decided to take hold of the situation. I was not going to let lung cancer take control of me. I called my hair stylist to set up an appointment to cut my hair as short as possible. He gave me a GI haircut.

A few days later, I was taking a shower. When I washed my hair, it came out by the handful. I looked in the mirror to see the extent of my loss. There was no hair on my head. Although this was a very emotional event, I felt a kind of relief. I could now focus on the big picture: "fighting the cancer." I breezed through my last treatment with little discomfort.

The doctors had warned me not to work because I would be too weak and tired to carry on with my full time job. However, I managed to work full-time, missing only the days of my chemotherapy treatments. Working helped maintain structure in what had become a chaotic life of doctor appointments and treatment. I felt that as long as I could work I would be okay. It helped take my mind off the disease.

Although loving people who supported me through this process surrounded me, my fear of how society felt about this disease did come true. One day I was grumbling about this disease and how tired and afraid I was. Someone overheard me and said, "If you didn't smoke, you would not be in this mess right now." I screamed back, "But I quit smoking three years ago. I don't deserve this disease, no one does."

In late August I returned to Boston for follow up. The doctors were very pleased at how well the tumors had responded to the chemotherapy and scheduled surgery for the first of September. I had my right lower lobe removed. I was in the hospital for nine days.

They sent the tissue to the pathologist, who said that the margins were clear. They also told me that there were no active tumors in the center of my chest. Once I healed from surgery, I would go on for my 25 rounds of radiation.

Radiation began in November. I went every day except Saturdays and Sundays. The treatment made me very tired and I slept a lot. Finally, in December, I was finished. I thought that I would bounce back as soon as it stopped, but I didn't. It took me several months before I started to regain my energy.

I was watching television while recovering at home one night. There was a program profiling several different cancer groups. Near the end of the segment, an organization called Alliance for Lung Cancer, Advocacy, Support, and Education was mentioned. I called the next day and joined their organization, which is now called Lung Cancer Alliance. I wanted to be a spokesperson for people with this disease. If anyone in Maine was diagnosed with lung cancer, I wanted to make sure that they had someone to talk with. I did not want them to have to go through this alone.

Since joining the Lung Cancer Alliance in 1999, I have become an advocate for the Dartmouth-Hitchcock Medical Oncology Board, and an Advocate for the Dana-Farber Cancer Institute. I have written proclamations declaring November as Lung Cancer

Awareness Month in Maine, which Governor Baldacci and former Governor King have signed.

I joined the American Association for Cancer Research in 2005. This organization's membership includes survivors and scientists who are dedicated to finding a cure for cancer. The annual meeting attracts over 16,000 scientists who come together from all over the world to share their research discoveries.

Progress is being made, but this disease is still deadly and could still happen to anyone. Although there are no tests to screen for lung cancer, there are some warning signs that should prompt medical attention. These include shortness of breath, a cough that does not go away, coughing up blood, fatigue, wheezing, chest, shoulder, back, or arm pain, repeated bouts of pneumonia or bronchitis, weight loss or loss of appetite, hoarseness, swelling of face of neck, general pain. So, if you or someone you know experiences any of these symptoms, please seek medical attention immediately. Finding this disease in its early stages is essential for long-term survival.

I continue to be closely monitored by the medical staff with CT scans, PET scans and X-rays. Once you have been diagnosed with this disease, it becomes a life-long journey of doctor appointments and tests. I am always on guard, wondering if my next appointment will put me back into treatment; or worse yet, if the cancer has come back in an area for which there is no hope for another remission. But, for the most part, I like to think that I have made lemonade out of the lemons that I received by turning my own personal challenges into helping make things better for others.

A resident of Augusta, Maine with a Graduate Degree in Public Health, the author is a passionate advocate for Lung Cancer research and awareness. She is a member of Lung Cancer Alliance, the American Association for Cancer Research, Dana-Farber Cancer Institute, and the Dartmouth-Hitchcock Medical Oncology Board.

An Unexpected Journey
Heather Saler

What had started out as a normal day ended up anything but. My grandmother had just passed away, I was a single mom and my 6-year-old son was away on vacation with his father. I was feeling stressed. While doing my daily treadmill workout, I developed mild heart palpitations. I stopped exercising, but the palpitations didn't stop. By that evening, my boyfriend of one year decided that a trip to the emergency room was in order. We entered the hospital, afraid there was a problem with my heart. Hours later, we walked out the door knowing the problem was in my lung. A CT scan the following morning led to more questions and more waiting. One week later, a CT-guided needle biopsy gave me my answer: I had non-small cell lung cancer, most likely Stage I.

I thought my entire world was ending. How could this be? I was only 33 and I'd never smoked. Lung cancer was not in my vocabulary! Surgery was suggested and I set out to find the best surgeon in town. Once I found him, I clung to his every word. Surgery gave me the best chance for a total cure. I was young, I was in overall good health, and I had caught it early. The doctor said that he would remove the cancer and I would return to my normal life.

The day before surgery, the Northeast was hit with a massive blizzard. When I called the hospital on the verge of hysteria, a kind staff member assured me that if I could make it in, the surgery would take place. At 4:00 a.m. the next morning, we shoveled our way out the front door to the car and traveled on snow-covered roads to make it to the hospital for my check-in time of 5:45 a.m. The last thing I recall before being put under is hearing the surgeon's voice as he walked into the room.

Surgery was difficult, but not as bad as I had imagined. I was up and walking the day after surgery, and sent home on the fourth day. I was fortunate to have the help and support of family and friends during the days when the simple act of sitting up felt like a full time job. Meals were taken care of, my son was taken to school and my every need was attended to.

I returned to the surgeon for my three-week follow up in good spirits. However, I was blindsided when I heard the following: "Your pathology report shows five mediastinal lymph nodes positive for cancer, which puts you at Stage IIIA. There is little hope that chemotherapy will increase your odds for survival." Those words echoed in my head. Was follow-up chemo useless, as the surgeon had said? Was I doomed? A panel of oncologists performed a further review of my records and recommended a regimen of daily radiation, along with weekly chemotherapy, for a period of six weeks. They felt this was my best shot at a cure.

The weekend before beginning my radiation regimen, my boyfriend proposed to me over a game of Scrabble by spelling out "Marry Me" on the board. His timing could not have been more perfect and I floated through the first few days of radiation on Cloud 9. However, as I was hooked up to my first chemo intravenous later that week, the seriousness of what I was up against finally hit me. From that day forward, I couldn't look at my son without crying. I would sit on his bed at night, watching him sleep as the tears flowed down my face. As I navigated my way through the unfamiliar territory of chemotherapy and radiation, each day began to feel worse than the next. The radiation treatment burned my esophagus and made it difficult to eat. The chemotherapy dehydrated me and I spent many afternoons hooked up to an I.V. receiving fluids. The nausea became constant, and I had to admit that I could no longer work. Each day that passed brought me closer to feeling that the end was imminent.

One night, while sitting on the edge of my son's bed watching him sleep, instead of crying and sadness, a fierce feeling of determination came over me. I *had* to make it through this treatment and beat this monster into submission. This little boy needed me and I needed him! That was the turning point in my treatment. I muddled through the remaining weeks—weak, dehydrated, nauseous and dizzy—but determined.

Treatment finally ended and I was thrilled to find that, despite my original fears, my life had not. As the days passed, I began to have more good moments than bad and I slowly began to feel human again. Month by month the lingering side effects lessened and I realized that there were a few moments during which I actually didn't think about cancer. My fiancé and I celebrated the one-year anniversary of my diagnosis by having a dream wedding onboard a cruise ship surrounded by close family and friends.

The months rolled by and I realized that while I was fortunate to have achieved remission, there are many thousands who do not. All of my research brought me to the conclusion that much more needs to be done to increase awareness and funding if we are ever going to bring about change. My husband and I decided to tackle a benefit walk, and the idea for "The First South Jersey Lung Cancer Walk/Run & Rally" was born. Our walk took place in November 2004, a beautiful, sunny Saturday morning, and we raised $32,000 for lung cancer research. Our second walk, held in November 2005, was an even greater success, raising over $45,000. Planning these events has been time consuming and often stressful, but worth every minute and I am so proud to play a small part in making a difference.

As I enter my third year post-diagnosis, I move forward with cautious optimism, putting one foot in front of the other, taking care of my body to the best of my ability with nutrition and exercise, nurturing my spiritual side and taking time each day to laugh.

It has been a bumpy ride, but one I would gladly repeat to have the same end result. I do not know where God plans to take me on this journey, but I wouldn't trade a moment of it. It has truly changed my life for the better and brought me a greater feeling of appreciation for all with which I am blessed.

A 37 year-old wife and mother, Heather was diagnosed with advanced stage lung cancer at the age of 33. Upon recovery, she stepped into the role of lung cancer advocate. In addition to speaking publicly to raise lung cancer awareness, she coordinates an annual lung cancer walk in New Jersey, raising donations for the *LUNGevity Foundation*, a national non-profit organization dedicated exclusively to funding innovative lung cancer research grants.

The Crystal Ball
Gail Matthews

In 2000, my husband and I were invited to Aspen, Colorado for our friend's inauguration as President of the American Medical Association. We danced at 11,000 feet above sea level and had a great time. After all the medical talk that evening, my husband suggested that we both fly to Cooper Clinic in Dallas to have a preventive heart scan EBT (Electronic Beam Topography). I told him not to waste his money on me, since I didn't feel I needed it. Well, he signed me up anyway. The test is simple, seven minutes from start to finish and you remain fully clothed. After the test, the radiologist told my husband he was fine, but to me he said, "Mrs. Matthews, you should get on a flight back to Boston and see a pulmonologist immediately. You have a spot on your lung. It could be inflammation, an infection or lung cancer." In a state of shock and disbelief, we canceled the rest of our plans and flew home. The next day I was with Dr. John Beamis, head of the Department of Pulmonary & Critical Care Medicine at Lahey Clinic in Burlington, Massachusetts.

Because I had no symptoms, lived a healthy life for all of my 60 years, ate well, stayed active and *never smoked*, he thought it was an infection, but ordered tests. I was prodded and poked with needles and everything came up negative. But the spot on my right lung remained and I was scheduled for an appointment with Dr. Christina Williamson, a lung surgeon. All of her tests were also negative, but she recommended that the spot be removed. A month later, after a second opinion by Dr. Doug Mathisen, head of Cardiology and Pulmonary Medicine at Massachusetts General Hospital, I scheduled surgery with Dr. Williamson. I chose December for the procedure, since it would allow my husband and me enough time to be home for Christmas and to go south for a few of the winter months. Also, I had just started the *Women Who Make a Difference*, a program for the Lake Sunapee Visiting Nurses Well Child Clinic and I wanted to complete the first one in 2000.

The surgeon found bronchial alveolar carcinoma and removed the lower lobe of my right lung. She took out ten lymph nodes for evaluation, found them free of cancer and declared me 95% cured. We got it early. After a painful, painful recovery I got better and was able to return to all of my normal activities, from horseback to bike riding.

In the spring of 2002, I found myself in the hospital with a stomach condition and dehydration. A routine X-ray detected a spot on my left lung. I reported this to Dr. Williamson and she immediately put me through CT scans, PET scans, bronchial tests, blood work and all the rest. The tests showed one spot on my lung and another at the base of my neck. It looked as if I would have to go through it all over again. In January 2003, they operated. Same thing: bronchial alveolar carcinoma and the lower left lobe was removed, but they found nothing at the base of my neck. More painful, painful recovery, but after a month I was riding my bike again, doing all of my activities and moving forward.

While in bed recovering from this second operation, I listened to the *Today Show*'s Katie Couric interview a young, well known actress. At the time I had no idea who she was but listened as she described her support for breast cancer research. She also seemed to say that she would never give her support to lung cancer research because she felt that those who get lung cancer deserve it. This was one of the very few times I cried, because I realized that the public perception was just that—you get lung cancer because you smoke. I *never smoked* and worked hard for the American Cancer Society in its anti-smoking campaigns. I thought I could get lots of things, but lung cancer wasn't one of them.

Well, I have learned a lot since the time of that interview. Then, I thought it was some sort of fluke for me to have gotten lung cancer. But I learned from Dr. David Sugarbaker at Brigham and Woman's Hospital in Boston that tall, white women who have never smoked are getting lung cancer at a higher rate than smokers and they don't know why. I fit that profile. I also learned that radon is the #2 cause of lung cancer and very little is known or done about that. The activist, proactive me was going to do some digging to find answers.

I asked Dr. Beamis why there was so little research on lung cancer going on. He told me that the dearth of funding had much to do with the stigma of smoking associated with the disease. I also learned that African Americans have the highest lung cancer mortality rate among Americans. In 2005, I learned that many young women and men in their 40's who had never smoked were being diagnosed with lung cancer.

After learning all of this, I decided to throw a ball to promote lung cancer awareness and to raise funds for research and for the Lung Cancer Alliance. Although as a volunteer I had founded the Reading, Massachusetts chapter of the American Cancer Society, where I worked on a no-smoking campaign in the workplace and public buildings, started a Cancer Registry, worked towards a Massachusetts spectrometer program for the public water system, helped get publicity for the Woburn Odor (Civil Action, a movie with John Travolta, became the story of the Woburn Odor) and founded "Love Lights a Tree" in New London, New Hampshire for the American Cancer Society, I felt that the ACS's focus on no-smoking campaigns did very little for the non-smoker who got cancer. Lung Cancer Alliance is the only national, non-profit organization dedicated solely to working on behalf of people living with or at risk for lung cancer.

The idea of the *Crystal Ball*, to clearly see the end of this disease, came to mind. We chose to hold the event in Boston and to honor seven top lung cancer doctors in the areas of surgery, research, and oncology. As of this writing, it is planned as a landmark event, to be attended by a growing group of philanthropic and corporate leaders and politicians from both parties, all of whom are committed to stopping the most lethal and misunderstood of all cancers. I have reached out to everyone to attend, to celebrate life and survivorship and to bring attention to a disease that, according to the U.S. Surgeon General, has reached epidemic proportions. My husband (the most supportive care giver and partner in the world) and I hired an event coordinator to help us on this and the seven doctors have told me they are thrilled to be a part of it. This has taken a lot of work since April of 2005, but the *Crystal Ball* will go on with God's help at the Copley Plaza in Boston. We have fabulous entertainment, including Boston's number one band, *White Heat*, and Misha Segal of Hollywood, an artist, composer and Emmy winner has donated his time for the event because his mom, his inspiration, died of lung cancer on Mother's Day. We need to do something to draw attention to the lack of funding and I know now that I am not alone.

Gail Matthews is a force of nature. The former Youth Fashion Director for a national retail apparel chain, she is a columnist for the *Boston Globe* and *The Hartford Times*, a former producer and host of a local television show, President of the Reading, New Hampshire Heart Association, founder of the Reading chapter of the American Cancer Society and founder of the Mammogram Fund for Women in Need. A resident of New Hampshire, Gail has been married for 47 years and she is the mother of two and the grandmother of six.

Editor's Note: The first-ever Crystal Ball, held in October, 2006 at the Copley Plaza Ballroom in Boston was a smashing success. Hosted by ABC News anchor Natalie Jacobsen and Boston Mayor Thomas Menino, the event raised over $120,000 for the Lung Cancer Alliance and featured guest speakers Dr. Deborah Morosini, sister of Dana Reeves, Billy Starr, who has raised over $200 million for cancer research through the Pan Mass Challenge, and awards for excellence to seven of the top cancer researchers in the Boston area.

Continued from page (54)

Talking with Your Doctor

Your physician has told you to make an appointment to discuss the results of your chest X-ray, CT scans and biopsy. Your initial impulse is to make that appointment as quickly as possible and hear the information that you are dreading to hear. It is critical to bring along to the appointment another set of eyes and ears, which could be your spouse, a relative, or even a friend who is closely interested in your medical care. Many studies have shown that the high level of stress associated with receiving unfavorable news about your diagnosis often results in your misunderstanding, not hearing, or simply not remembering the vast majority of the information given to you by the physician. Ask your companion to listen attentively and take notes, or even, with the physician's permission, record the conversation. That will enable your companion to help answer any questions you have in the days following the consultation.

When calling to make the appointment, tell the receptionist that your doctor wants to see you for some very serious and important news and you would like to know if it would be possible to schedule you as the last appointment of the day. Why? Because your best chance of getting the doctor to block out sufficient time to answer all of your questions and concerns in a relaxed and unrushed manner is to make sure that he does not have patients waiting to see him after your conference. The receptionist or office manager will most likely check with the physician and this will remind him that he will be having a very sensitive discussion with you. If he cannot schedule your appointment at the end of his patient schedule, he may at least carve out a sufficient amount of time during the day so that he can give you all of his attention, undisturbed.

Continued on page (88)

How I Met My Mother
(and How She Met Me)
Susan Levin

My mother's diagnosis of lung cancer was a curse, but also a gift. Before her diagnosis we were not especially close: my mother was, first and foremost, my late father's wife. There was always a distance between us—in part it was generational, in part, the "normal" distance experienced by many children of immigrants. Chasia (Ida in English), was always second-in-command and often rather subservient to her strong-willed husband. It was not until she was diagnosed with lung cancer and I moved in with her that I came to regard her as someone extremely special, a true woman of valor. The days we spent together during her illness made me realize just how much I loved my mother. For her part, as she told me before she died, she never expected that I would put my life on hold to be with her. Because of lung cancer, we came to share an extraordinary gift; we truly came to love each other as only a mother and daughter can.

Both of my parents were Holocaust survivors. I was born and had lived in Germany until I was three years old. At some point, I came to identify the survival tactics my parents had to learn. Their suffering made them very self-reliant. They believed they could endure anything. They never complained and never allowed anyone else to do so. They were not very trusting and often kept outsiders at a distance. While they never asked for anyone's help, they were quick to give theirs. Like so many of their survivor friends, they got married as soon as the war was over and within a few years had a child, me. Despite the horrors of the camps, they made a commitment to building a new life together. The only time they were apart was when one of them was in the hospital.

My father, whom I loved dearly, suffered a heart attack at home and simply refused to go to the hospital. True to his character, he believed he could overcome what he called "this sort of heart attack." He felt that if he could survive being chained to an electrified fence, as he had been during the war, he could survive anything. He refused to let my mother call an ambulance. Though the pain was excruciating, he had to handle the emergency in his own way. This determination led to congestive heart failure and he passed away ten months later. It was his strength of will that kept him alive for those ten months; the doctors were truly astounded.

My mother was devastated after my father died but decided life was still worth living. She resumed her volunteer activities and became even more active in the community. Difficult as it was after the end of her fifty years of marriage, she was successful until she began experiencing some of the typical but often vague symptoms of lung cancer: shortness of breath and chest pain. First a chest X-ray (they thought it was pneumonia), then a PET scan followed by a needle biopsy, a bone scan and other tests. Finally a diagnosis that shocked us: lung cancer.

We thought that was impossible. Like so many others, we associated lung cancer with smoking. How could my mother, neither a smoker nor someone overly exposed to second-hand smoke, have lung cancer? We learned the hard way that you do not have to be a smoker to get lung cancer. One in five women diagnosed with lung cancer never smoked. Like so many others, my mother's lung cancer was diagnosed in its latter stages when the disease is inoperable and potentially incurable. The doctor's recommendation was a course of chemotherapy, which is not a cure but does prolong life and even enables one to live a fairly "normal" life for as long as the drugs work. For my mother, that was almost eighteen months.

After her diagnosis, I sold my apartment in Manhattan and moved in with her, crossing the border to New Jersey. My mother did not want me to live with her. She felt she was ruining my life and, likewise, she did not want to appear dependent. For me, there were many adjustments. I became the chauffeur, since my mother never learned to drive a car. She would not hear of hiring a cleaning person. The Holocaust mentality reared up: hire someone to do your dirty work, unheard of! This was her home and only she could take care of it! A turning point in our relationship came when she decided I could clean her house. As much as I did not relish the thought, I quickly realized that allowing me to clean her house was my mother's way of reaching out to me. Soon enough, she gave me a closet for my clothes and even acknowledged to her friends that I was living with her.

Those were the little things. What was really important was that, for the first time, my mother and I would actually talk, about the past as well as the present and the future. She was very concerned about my future. She wanted me to date and get married. She was constantly worried that I would be alone. My mother's every waking thought was not about herself, but about others. We discussed literature and politics and we gossiped, all the things we never did before. I began not only to like and respect my mother but to truly love her for the person she was: a wonderful, funny, special human being, someone I might never have known were it not for her diagnosis of lung cancer.

Gradually, her disease took more and more of her energy and spirit away. When it came to the point that she could not tie her own shoelaces and could not manage her beloved needlepoint, she decided it was time to go. My mother wanted to join her husband.

She asked me to call her best friend to say good bye. She also asked that I call the rabbi of the synagogue. It was time for the final prayers.

Even in the final days of her life, her first thoughts were about others. She was concerned that if she died on the "wrong day" it would spoil the Bat Mitzvah of her grand niece. I truly believe she made sure to die on Friday so that her funeral would be on Sunday, allowing the celebration to go on as planned.

When she passed, I felt overwhelming grief and guilt. How could I have missed out on what a special person my mother was for all those years? How could I have overlooked her kindness and generosity? I am deeply sorry for what she suffered but if she hadn't been diagnosed with the disease I might never have learned how exceptional she was. All those special moments we enjoyed together might never have happened.

Because of the experience with my mother and because I did not want other families to be surprised by a diagnosis of lung cancer like we had been, together with others I founded the Lung Cancer Circle of Hope in January of 2006. Our mission is to educate the public, including the medical community, about lung cancer, the disease, which is not synonymous with smoking, the addiction, a fact of which many are not aware. All that I am doing to raise awareness of lung cancer is in memory of the incredible woman whom I called Mommy.

The legislation proclaiming every November Lung Cancer Awareness Month in New Jersey was introduced in memory of my mother. Our educational symposia, entitled *Lung Cancer: Dispelling the Myths, Dispensing the Facts* are presented at various locations around the state. We are working with local, county and state government officials to promote a greater understanding of the #1 cancer killer of men and women. While I certainly wish it had happened in a different way, my mother's lung cancer diagnosis gave us both opportunities that we might otherwise not have had. We both got to know and love each other as never before. We both grew as human beings and I am a much better person for the experience.

Susan Levin is the Founder and President of the Lung Cancer Circle of Hope, a non-profit corporation the mission of which is to educate the public, the medical community and public policy makers about lung cancer. She is a member of New Jersey's Lung Cancer Work Group of the State Comprehensive Cancer Plan, the Research Advocates Network, the National Lung Cancer Partnership and the Cancer Control and Prevention Advisory Group. She resides in Lakewood, New Jersey.

Part III
TAKING CHARGE

Healing takes courage, and we all have courage, even if we have to dig a little to find it.

—*Tori Amos*

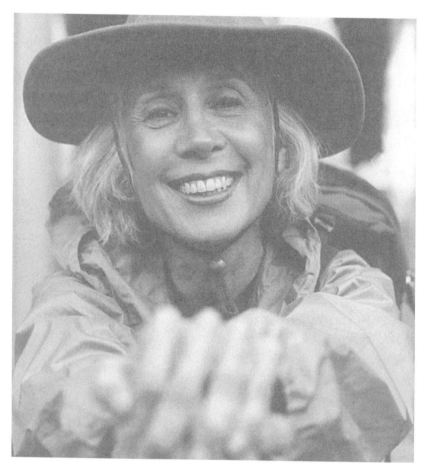

Dee Redfearn, page 239

It's All In the Odds:
The Surprising Journey of a
Multiple Cancer Victim
William Jones

In 1998 I had open-heart surgery and in a roundabout way this led to my being diagnosed with a slow-growing prostate cancer. My doctor recommended the "wait and see" approach, working under the assumption that I would die of other causes long before the prostate cancer would claim me. For insurance, he began administering a hormone to retard the growth of the cancer. My prostate cancer was monitored regularly, with no indication that the cancer had grown or spread.

Two years later, I experienced blood in my urine. This had happened before and each time it proved to be from my prostate problems. This time, my urologist suggested a CT scan, just to play it safe. The scan detected a tumor in my bladder, which subsequent surgery revealed to be an invasive, aggressive form of bladder cancer. I received mixed recommendations about treatment from my long-term urologist and from two different oncologists. I was particularly concerned with their seeming lack of urgency about my future course.

Confused and apprehensive, I contacted a major cancer institute. After a comprehensive examination, its oncologist laid out my options. It became obvious that for me to have a reasonable chance of survival I would need to have at least a portion of my bladder removed. Several days later, I met with the institute's urologist, who would determine both the extent of the surgery needed and stage of the cancer, which would determine if and to what extent the cancer may have spread.

Part of the pre-operative procedure called for a scan to check for other cancers. The technician told me that there would be a single pass of the scanning equipment. However, after the first scan, they had me remain on the table. They then made several more scans. I was sure they had found something, but I was told everything was normal and that the radiologist would review the test and give the results to my doctor.

My urologist told me that the CT scan had disclosed a suspicious spot on the upper right lobe of my lung. An appointment was made for a needle biopsy to determine if the spot was benign or malignant.

At the hospital the following Monday, I was ushered into still another CT scanning facility. I was told that long needles would be inserted into my chest cavity from different angles to, hopefully, obtain tissue samples from the spot. The procedure had several risks, the major one being a chance that it could collapse my lung. Worried, I laid back on the hard scanning table and watched as they pressed the long needles into my chest. The procedure seemed to go on forever. Then suddenly everything stopped. Minutes later, the doctors reappeared. My lung had collapsed, and, worst of all, they had been unable to get a sample for the pathologist. I would be taken to a hospital room for the afternoon, where one of the needles in my chest would be attached to a suction device to suck out the air and re-inflated my lung. I was told this was quite routine, but I was scared.

The painful biopsy procedure was repeated. When it was over, I could see the staff talking and gesturing. My lung had collapsed again, but fortunately this time they thought they might have gotten a usable sample.

Back in a hospital room, they hooked up the suction equipment to a small tube in the front of my chest and began sucking out the air. I was self-conscious, lying on my back on the hospital bed when I felt so healthy. It seemed so ridiculous. Still, I had no choice. They were the doctors and I assumed they knew what they were doing. I was supposed to hear the results the following morning, a Wednesday. It still wasn't clear to me if they had been able to obtain a usable tissue sample.

Thursday morning arrived with still no results. I demanded my biopsy report. Later that morning, my oncologist informed me that I had a third, primary cancer, lung cancer. I was too shocked, too disturbed, and too furious to even question her.

I had confused and conflicting reactions to the news. I knew that all cancers were potentially life threatening. I had by then read enough about prostate and bladder cancer to know a little about them. Oh, I still had many questions about them. For example, how would I urinate if I no longer had a bladder? But now, I had still another cancer to think about, one about which I knew absolutely nothing. Over the next two days, no nurse or doctor came to my room. I demanded information about my lung cancer, but I was told repeatedly that only my doctor was allowed to answer my questions.

Finally, on the second afternoon, a nurse appeared, angrily demanding to know why I was making such a disturbance. By then, I was so gripped by emotion that I had difficulty even speaking. Through tear-filled eyes, sobbing bitterly, I explained my frustration. Patiently she stood, listening to my anguish. When I stopped, she turned around without a word and strode from the room.

Minutes later, a beautiful young woman came into my room. The nurse introduced her as Dr. Bibyack, the pulmonary resident on the floor. The young doctor explained to me that she had been monitoring my case, and that everything that had been done was appropriate and according to common medical practice. She went on to explain that there were different types of lung cancer. She informed me that the cancer I had was usually treated by surgical removal, in my case, of the upper right lobe of my lung. She told me that that lobe represented approximately one quarter of my total lung capacity. She described the incision, a lengthy one under my right arm, accessed by spreading the ribs open. It was a major surgical procedure requiring a lengthy hospitalization.

When this lovely young lady left, I felt an overwhelming sense of relief. I was resolved to undergo still another major operation. But most of all there was indescribable relief from knowing, understanding more about this cancer. She had treated me with respect, as an intelligent person, and left me with the sense that someone in this hospital really cared for and respected me.

When the young doctor was in my room answering my questions, the nurse had remained at my side. After the doctor left, she placed her hand gently on my shoulder and said, "Mr. Jones, you are a very sick man!" I have never been so affected by words. I had experienced absolutely no pain since the large tube had been driven into my chest that first evening. Physically I had never felt better. And still, here was the reality that I had three different, deadly cancers. I had been in denial. This, the hand on my shoulder and the words, were reality, a defining moment.

The following morning, the urologist explained the surgical options that I had for my abdominal surgery, explained the operation to me, and answered all my questions. I accepted his recommendations. I was in control now, making decisions on my care and treatment.

Early Wednesday morning I was wheeled to the operating room. I was astonished to learn later that I was in surgery for more than eight-and-a-half hours. The pathology report on the prostate cancer that had been removed along with my bladder showed that it had become immune to the hormone treatment and had spread through much of my prostate. The cancer had been removed just in time.

I went home after 23 days in the hospital with multiple tubes in my body. In the weeks that followed, the bandages were replaced, the tubes flushed and finally removed. I was returning to a normal existence, my new, synthetic bladder operating perfectly.

Then it became a furious race against time to regain my strength for the removal of my lung lobe before that cancer spread. I worked very hard, exercising and walking at the local rehabilitation center. In no time, I was walking two miles a day on the treadmill and lifting heavy weights.

Some six weeks after my abdominal surgery, I underwent what had been described to me as routine pre-surgical pulmonary tests. One of my sons and my wife accompanied me and afterwards we were led into the doctor's conference room. Presumably, we were there to schedule a date for my surgery. But when the doctor finally came in, I knew by the look on his face that there was a problem: the results of my pulmonary tests precluded the surgery, my only chance for survival. I was utterly devastated.

The following week at the rehabilitation center where I was working out to regain my strength, I tearfully recounted my story to a young psychologist. She told me that I wasn't depressed, but that I was suffering from a perfectly understandable case of severe anxiety. I found myself pouring out my life story to her in a flood of uncontrolled emotions. Afterwards, I felt guilty at having revealed so much of my innermost feelings and thoughts to this total stranger. However, at that same moment, somehow everything changed. Life took on a new meaning.

I rushed home, desperate and determined. I phoned my oncologist. She confirmed that she had spoken with my surgeon, and agreed that surgery was not an option. I tried to make it clear that I would accept any risk, including death on the operating table, to avoid certain death from the cancer. Desperate, I asked her to arrange for another CT scan, hoping that I could use it to support my efforts. She agreed.

The following morning, a Saturday, the doorbell rang. It was Dr. Hannam, our family physician for some thirty years who had come at my request. He listened while I pleaded my case for surgery. He gave me a physical examination and promised to phone my thoracic surgeon the following Monday. I was so appreciative: here was the needed ray of hope.

The following Monday, I received a phone call from Dr. Hannam, who assured me the surgeon would perform the surgery and that he would be calling me. Three days later the surgeon's office called to confirm that he would perform the surgery. He had talked with my pulmonary doctor, who would decide on the date of surgery, when he felt I was strong enough to undergo the procedure.

I can't describe the relief I felt at that moment. I had received a gift of life! I could not believe my good fortune. I was scheduled to have my CT scan later that same day. I debated canceling it, but I decided to have it, just in case I might need it to help my cause.

The day after the CT scan, my oncologist told me that the cancer had nearly doubled in size in just two months. It was critical that I have the surgery as soon as possible. But there was another problem. The scan had disclosed a suspicious spot on my adrenal gland, one of the most common areas to which lung cancer spreads. They would have to take a needle biopsy the next day. Suddenly, my life's roller coaster was headed downhill again.

The following morning I received a call from the pathology department with the news that the spot on my adrenal gland was benign. When I was wheeled into the operating room it was filled with people all busily rushing about. The room was icy cold. Three hours later, I was moved into intensive care. My surgeon told my wife that everything could not have gone more perfectly. She recalls how happy, even delighted the surgeon seemed to be.

I went home ten days later. I had my final appointment with my thoracic surgeon weeks after the surgery. He welcomed me with a hug. He admitted that he had at first refused to perform the operation. But he described his lengthy discussion with Dr. Hannam, after which he had come to have a real respect for him. It was Dr. Hannam who had persuaded him to go forward with the surgery. He told of days of worry and regret for having made the commitment to operate. He described writing out a long list of all that could go wrong and corrective actions. Ecstatically, he claimed that all his fears and concerns were for naught and that he could not believe how well I had recovered. I was his living reward. He is a great man.

The human body is an incredible machine, becoming more efficient when portions are removed, but hardly capable of fully compensating for the loss of a quarter of the lung's capacity. I am breathing without the need for supplementary oxygen, even at night. I am a five-year prostate, bladder and lung cancer survivor. I have examined the odds of my cancers. They are pretty favorable for prostate and bladder cancers. But the five year survival rate of all males with lung cancer is 12.4%. I realize how fortunate I am just to be here!

The author is the retired Program Manager for Space Shuttle Redesign for the Thiokol Corporation. At 82, He is an active participant in Wisconsin lung cancer advocacy programs promoting lung cancer education, early screening and improved services at local clinics and hospitals and has been a featured guest on local television health news reports.

Continued from page (72)

Choosing the Right Doctor

How do you judge whether your physician or the specialist who made the diagnosis and who may be in charge of your treatment is the right healthcare professional to manage your disease? She will give you this uncomfortable news as follows: you and your companion will come into her office or a small empty hospital conference room; she will close the door and sit four to six feet from you at eye level. The doctor will first ask for your thoughts about your medical situation and how you size it up. After you answer, she will tell you that she has reviewed your file, gone over all of the laboratory information and medical imaging tests, spoken with the necessary consultants and that she has some serious or difficult news to give you. She will tell you that you have a diagnosis of lung cancer that was made on the basis of all the medical information that has been collected about your case. She will then pause to give you some time to absorb the news and react. Your reaction could be anything, from intent listening, to crying, anger, fear, guilt or a range of other emotions. When the physician sees that you have recovered somewhat, more explanations will follow. She will explain that, while the diagnosis is serious, there are treatments that can either eliminate or control the disease and afford you a longer and better quality of life. Ideally, the physician will talk to you in a slow, soft, sympathetic manner, giving you and your companion the opportunity to ask questions at any time, all of which she will answer in a calm, easy-to-understand manner. The physician will have taken steps to minimize interruptions such as beepers and telephone calls. She may offer to have you come back at another time or contact her by telephone with additional questions.

The physician who tells you about the diagnosis may be your family practitioner or internist and it may not be the physician who treats your illness; it therefore may not be possible for him to go into detail about your therapy regimen. It is important to keep in mind, however, that your internist or family practitioner will remain an important part of your healthcare team. If the physician has presented this difficult news in the fashion that I described, you will want to see him on a regular basis. Even if he does nothing more than talk to you, he will keep tabs on your other, peripheral medical problems and explain to you what the treating physicians are doing. That way, you will be informed of communications between your doctors. At this stage, it is extremely important not to abandon your personal physician simply because he may not be the doctor treating your lung cancer.

Continued on page (106)

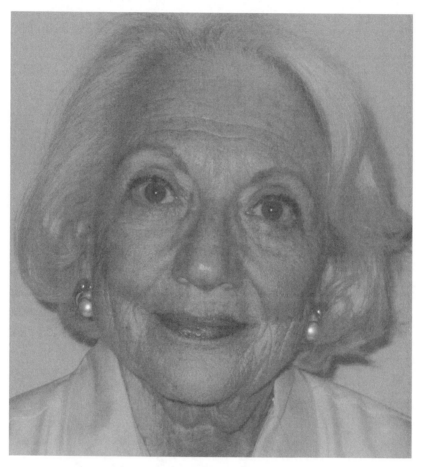

Marvelle Colby, page 91

Got Cancer? Consider This!

Marvelle S. Colby

In November 2000, I was diagnosed with non-small cell lung cancer, which, in my case, once it metastasizes, has a 1% five-year survival rate. After treatment on a total of seven tumors—four lung tumors, two neck tumors and a brain tumor—by four conventional surgeries and one stereotactic radio surgery using a powerful, computer-directed radiation beam, and after several courses of conventional radiation, I am now cancer free. The notes in my medical records refer to the "unusual course" of my cancer. I asked my oncologist what this meant and he told me the unusual aspect was that I was still alive.

Am I unique? Or am I just lucky? Is it a miracle, or the ability of a gifted doctor who incorporates complementary and alternative evidence-based medicine (CAM) in his practice that allows me to live?

In January 2001, I underwent surgery to remove what appeared to be a small tumor confined to the lower left lobe of the lung. The surgeon noticed something in the upper left lobe, which she also removed. That "something" turned out to be a form of lung cancer so small it hadn't shown up on any scans. I spent almost two weeks in the hospital after the surgery. When I returned for my six-week check-up, I reported a most bothersome cough.

A short time later, I noticed what appeared to be a swollen gland beneath the jawbone on the right side of my face. I went to my primary physician, who sent me for a CT scan, which revealed not a swollen gland, but a tumor. My doctor referred me to a neck surgeon at the same hospital I had left just two months before. A biopsy determined that this new tumor had metastasized from that small, almost unseen tumor in the upper left lobe of my lung that had been found and removed during my last surgery.

Preparing for yet another operation required a PET scan, which revealed not only the metastasized neck tumor, but also a brain tumor. Doctors #3 and #4, a radiologist and a neurologist, removed the brain tumor using stereotactic radio surgery. Doctor #5, the neck surgeon, removed the neck tumor. Doctor #6, a dentist, saw me to ensure that my teeth were in good enough condition to withstand radiation. Doctor #7, a second radiation oncologist, managed the follow-up radiation.

While recovering from all this and five months from the original surgery, I noticed yet another swelling, this time under my chin. It hurt and kept getting bigger and bigger. Pretty soon it was the size of a grapefruit, covering the lower jawbone on the left side of my face. To Doctor #8, an oncologist, I reported that the neck surgeon had told me, over and over during an office visit and in repeated phone calls, that this was in the neck surgeon's opinion merely a "radiation wattle," a reaction to the radiation I had received.

The oncologist ordered another CT scan, which revealed the growth to be yet another tumor. Having been allowed to grow unchecked and untreated for six weeks, the latest tumor—the fifth so far—was inoperable. I requested a different neck surgeon, Doctor #9. She was not confident, also concerned that the tumor was inoperable and that, even if it were, I might very well need skin grafts to my face and neck. It was decided to reduce the tumor to an operable size with radiation. So it was back to Doctor #7, the radiation oncologist, whom I had come to trust.

It was at this juncture, facing five more weeks of radiation to hopefully reduce the size of the tumor, that I considered leaving this highly rated hospital. If this was the best that generally accepted medicine had to offer in dealing with cancer, I thought it might be wise to consider medical treatment outside the mainstream.

I realize now that I was moving from being a passive to an active participant in my battle with cancer. I requested copies of all my records and began researching my options for something beyond surgery, radiation, and chemotherapy. With this information in hand, I started my radiation treatment, but made an appointment to see a new, special doctor. Exploring the literature on complementary and alternative medicine I learned that common practice is not always the best practice. My search led me to a doctor who was a board certified internist, but who practices "evidence-based medicine"—the use of current best evidence in making medical decisions about individual patients—and whose medical abilities reached far beyond that of most conventional physicians. The treatments he frequently prescribed included a specific diet, off-label medicine, Chinese herbs that enhance the immune system and various vitamins and supplements.

I told this new doctor I wanted to strengthen my immune system to withstand the radiation and surgery yet to come. In addition to medications, he prescribed a special diet and a regimen of Chinese herbs which he had personally formulated. One of the drugs he suggested to treat cancer was looked upon with some skepticism by mainstream medicine at the time but has since become more widely accepted. One of the medications he prescribed lowered my white blood count, so he changed the dosage. Other than that, none of these medications or supplements has had any negative side effects.

Given my unanticipated recovery and sudden end to what had been rapidly occurring metastases, it is clear to me that the regimen had a most positive effect. All of this was done not instead of, but as a complement to the customary, conventional treatment.

While I was under active treatment, the hospital doctors were kept informed of this alternative treatment, just as my internist was informed of theirs.

The removal of the fifth tumor went remarkably well. The radiation had reduced the size of the tumor and Doctor #7 managed to implant radioactive seeds in my neck as part of the same operation. The surgeon projected a ten-day to two-week hospital stay. To the surprise of my hospital physicians, I tolerated the procedure so well I was sent home in two days. I am convinced this was due to the benefits of the complementary treatment I had received. The rapid metastasis had ceased and there were no new tumors!

That is, until October, 2004, when my oncologist reported a change in my CT scan. Back in 2001, he saw spots on my right lung. I knew that each time I had a follow-up CT scan the possibility of a change was lurking, and now it had happened. But the oncologist said, "Go to Florida for the winter as you planned. The scans make 'slices' and it's possible this isn't a change but just a shadow caused by the angle of the scan." I looked at him horrified. There was no way I could relax and enjoy the sunny South. My mind wouldn't let me.

I called the surgeon and asked her to review the latest scan. She did and said, "Let's be sure." A needle biopsy was ordered and the news was "Yes, it's cancer." "Get it out," I said, and in November of 2004 she operated and removed two benign and two new primary lung tumors in the upper and middle lobes of my right lung. Yes, I did go to Florida, a little later than planned, and much relieved. Relieved because after the surgery, I saw my special doctor and his words were "You're lucky." Having the oncologist tell me that there was a high possibility of reoccurrence, I didn't feel especially lucky. Having had seven tumors and yet another hospital stay, even another successful surgery didn't make me feel lucky.

But he meant lucky in another way. A new treatment, based on programmed cell death, was now available. He prescribed another investigational drug. Again I signed all the legal releases, and again I was able to receive this new medicine on a compassionate use basis.

Today, almost six years since that fateful diagnosis in November 2000, I continue to be a survivor of Stage IV metastatic non-small cell lung cancer. Yes, when I bend over or climb hills I do become short of breath. Nevertheless, I enjoy my family and friends and regularly swim half a mile, work out at a fitness center, walk two miles, line dance weekly, and sing in two choirs, all of which, I believe, increase my lung capacity. I returned to work briefly and retired at age seventy.

By adding to my medical team an extraordinary medical practitioner who understands that conventional medicine does not yet have all the answers, I believe I have extended and enhanced the quality of my life. Most of the doctors know my special doctor, a former colleague of theirs at the hospital. I sense the beginnings of openness among mainstream caregivers to CAM. The neurologist does ask about the special doctor's treatment and at one follow-up visit, she asked me for his card.

No one knows how long my lung cancer will be held at bay. That includes all nine members of the team of cancer specialists treating me at one of the world's best known cancer centers. We should all be aware that clinical trials and medical research are concurrently underway where scientists are researching outcome-based therapies and approaches. Many researchers are reporting on success with new uses of existing drugs in treating cancers. Some of these modalities have proven beneficial in preventing and fighting illness, but have fallen outside the standard protocols of mainstream medical practice and are not widely in use.

My experience has convinced me of the absolute need for the patient to take an informed and active role in any treatment decisions. The conventional cancer care I continue to receive at the hospital, complemented by the care I received from an "out of the box" practitioner has resulted in my case being labeled by the oncologist as "unusual", in this case, a happy outcome.

Dr. Colby is Emeritus Professor of Management at Marymount Manhattan College where she taught for 25 years following 15 years of diverse management experience in the for profit, public, and non-profit sectors, including service as the Florida Regional Manager for the Washington, D.C.- based Center for Human Services, Chairperson of the Dade County Commission on the Status of Women and Executive Director of the Girl Scout Council of Greater New York. She has authored and/or co-authored three books. Her significant contributions have been recognized by her election to the Hunter College Hall of Fame and to Marquis' Who's Who in America. When her illness became known to her students, alumni, and colleagues, The Dr. Marvelle S. Colby Endowed Scholarship Fund was established. The fund of over $100,000 will underwrite the education of financially disadvantaged business management students at Marymount.

You Cannot Tell Live From Dead!

Natalie Smith Parra

My cancer was diagnosed five and a half years ago, a barely noticed mass on a routine chest X-ray. A nurse paged me when I was shopping; I had to go outside to call her from a pay phone. "There's a mass on your left lung," the nurse said. "Can you come in for a CT scan this afternoon, before 5:30?" I agreed to go. I didn't really know what a mass on the lung meant, nor exactly how a CT scan worked.

The first scan took place in a windowless room of the hospital basement. I lay on the table while the doctor injected dye into a bulging vein in the crook of my arm. The radiologist came out from behind an enclosure. He spoke to me softly, "What are you here for?" he asked me. "I'm not sure," I said. "Something about a mass on my lung."

Later, as I was leaving, he wished me good luck. I smiled and shrugged. I was thirty-eight years old. I still felt the invincibility of youth. I was not yet too worried about this "mass" which, I figured, would be cleared up with some kind of pill.

The next time, the nurse called me at home. "Natalie, there's definitely a mass there. It looks pretty small, about 2 centimeters."

"That's good, isn't it?" I asked. "Is it cancer?" "It could be cancer," she said cautiously, "but it could be some kind of infection."
She made an appointment for me with a thoracic surgeon for the
following Thursday.

In the surgeon's waiting room, a tall young resident with an
Eastern European accent introduced himself. He asked a lot of
questions and jotted down my answers. "Wait, wait," I held up
my hand. "Aren't we here to talk about options? Tests, biopsies or
something? The nurse told me that you could take a sputum sample with a bronchoscope. How about that?" The doctor shook his
head. "Bronchoscopies are for people I don't want to operate on.
You have a small mass. We'll remove it."

The resident explained the surgery to me. In three weeks they
would perform a thoracotomy, opening my thorax by cutting
through the rib cage. What happened after that would depend on
what the surgeon saw inside. The resident set up an appointment
for my pre-operative blood work.

The operation was supposed to take four or five hours; when my
family saw the surgeon step out of the elevator after only two
hours, they thought I was dead. He motioned for them to sit in an
alcove in the corner of the waiting room. He told them that the
mass was cancer and that it had spread to lymph nodes throughout my chest. Taking out the lung wouldn't help, so he just closed
me back up. He would refer me to an oncologist, he said; maybe
there was some treatment for me, but he doubted it. He suggested
that my family not discuss any of this with me.

I woke up in the recovery room, my bed the last in a row of seven
or eight. At first, the lights were so bright I could only squint. I
looked down the row and felt some relief that the stiff white sheets
were pulled up only to the other patients' chins: I knew I wasn't
in the morgue. My head felt heavy, thick with morphine. My eyes
strained to focus and finally found the surgeon, sitting next to my
mother seated on chairs against the wall. My mother's arms were

crossed, her lips pressed tight. Her face betrayed her exhaustion. I noticed on the hospital tray next to me a brochure on hospice care. Although the doctor saw me trying to focus, he ignored me and said to my mother. "She could go to hospice for pain," he said. "I didn't have any pain until this operation," I said. He let out a short laugh.

I drew my veil of denial tight around me. I wouldn't accept his prognosis. I couldn't: I had a four-year-old child to raise, eleventh grade students to teach, and a world to change. I was supposed to die a happy old woman.

Soon after my release from the hospital, my mother, my sister and I drove across town to a large university hospital center for an appointment with an oncologist, an expert on lung cancer and cancers of unknown origin. She would give us a second opinion on the kind of therapy I should receive.

Across from us behind a big desk the doctor silently flipped through my file, paused where something interested her, then flipped some more. My sister pulled from her bag a bouquet of Tootsie Pops, orange, purple, red, brown and offered one to the doctor. "Oh, yeah, thanks," the doctor said, reaching across the desk. "Sugar is my weakness." She chose the red one and swirled it around inside her mouth as she talked. "Well," she said, "your cancer is Stage III." I nodded.

She recommended chemotherapy: Taxol and Carboplatin. My lawyer sister popped a chocolate sucker into her mouth. "Listen, I've been thinking," she said pointing her Tootsie Pop at the doctor. "I say, if that's the recommended amount, we double it. The more the better, the way I see it. Let's be aggressive here." The doctor's eyes grew wide, "I don't want to kill your sister," she said and smiled. "How many people with this disease have you cured?" I asked. The doctor looked down and let out her breath, her knuckles whitened on the edges of the folder. "No one," she said. I shouldn't have asked. I already knew the answer. I'd known it for a month now, since I woke up in the white glow of the recovery room lights.

Soon after, I began eighteen long weeks of chemotherapy treatments. My first day, a nurse rubbed her thumb over the back of my hand. "You have good veins," she said. My mother stood at the door and watched the nurse hang the first slick bag of Taxol. The oncologist came in, wearing her white coat with a name patch and ink stains on the pocket. She placed my file on a counter. I saw a hexagonal yellow sticker on the file emblazoned with black letters: "Interesting Case: Do Not Discard."

Before treatments began, I had contacted an organization about a retreat for cancer patients. Twice during my chemotherapy the administrator returned my call, to find out if I was interested in participating. I had my children tell her I wasn't home. I just didn't feel like talking to anyone. Then, luckily, the third time she called, I picked up the phone.

"Listen," she said. "I don't want you to take that surgical opinion as a death sentence."

"Uh, okay. Whatever."

"I have the phone number of a very good lung surgeon." She said. "Maybe you should make an appointment."

"Okay. Thank you." I took more Ativan and went back to sleep.

She called the next morning, but I shook my head: "tell her I'm not here," I motioned to my son. At that point, stoned on Ativan, the only position I could tolerate was curled into a ball in a dark room, my face buried in a cool pillow. No sight, no sound, no light. I was like a fetus who twists and twitches itself into the birth position, readying itself for life, except that I was preparing for death.

All hope was gone. I was not accepting death well. There was nothing left to rage against, nothing to fight. My body had betrayed me and the disease would win. I felt none of the peace associated with being near the so-called "other side". I wanted to buy my four-year-old daughter a winter coat for every year I wouldn't be with her, but that wouldn't do. She would need so much more.

The retreat lady called again. I told her I was sick of doctors poking me and looking at me as if I were already dead. I told her I had run out of energy for doctors. "Please, Natalie," she implored. "What can one more appointment hurt? I thought about her question. "No," I said. I appreciate your concern, but I don't think I can do it."

My mother disagreed. "We might as well go. That way, if he says no too, we'll know we did all we could." We went. The new surgeon was unhappy with the CT films I brought from the HMO. He clucked his tongue. "They didn't even use contrast," he said. In addition to a suitable CT scan, he ordered an MRI of the brain, a bone scan and a PET scan to rule out distant metastasis. He also ordered my first mediastinoscopy—a biopsy of the lymph nodes of the trachea. If there was no cancer in the lymph nodes on the right side of my trachea, the doctor explained, I would be able to have surgery. If successful, my chances of surviving until the end of the year would jump from less than five percent to around thirty-five percent. It was my best hope, my last real chance. The mediastinoscopy would determine if surgery would be appropriate. I passed all the other tests. I waited for the results of the trachea test.

A week after the procedure, I watched my four year old daughter, oblivious to my tortured waiting, kick up sparkling shards of water at her swim class. I stepped outside the class to check my messages. One was from Dr. Scott, the new surgeon. His voice was excited. He had good news. We could schedule the surgery, he said. I cried as I fumbled to dial his number.

"The pathology report shows no evidence of disease in any of your lymph nodes," he said, "not even on the left side. What the other doctor saw on the films was just dead tissue." "By the way," he added, "the HMO has to pay for the operation."

On the day of my surgery, before the July heat began to broil the city, Dr. Scott opened my chest and removed my whole left lung. Then he gently sliced the thin membrane under which lay my beating heart and scraped away the tumor that had attached itself to my aorta.

The morning after the surgery, my doctor pulled a chair to the side of my bed. "The operation was a success," he said. We sat and smiled at each other for a few minutes, both shaking our heads in disbelief. He told me he had removed my left lung and that the tumor around my aorta was already hard and dead, like dry clay.

"I touched it with a scalpel," he said, "and it fell right off. Dead tissue."

"Why did the old doctor tell me nothing had changed?" I ask.

"He just looked at the CT films, which can show both live and dead tissue," he explained. That's why, in cases like this, you need a biologic sample. You had an excellent response to the chemotherapy."

It isn't a cure, he reminded me. Cancer is tricky, but he was optimistic. He will watch me closely for the next five years. Five years, five years, five years—like an incantation. I am sure that number will always be dancing in my head. But I wake up these days glad to be alive and with a newfound love of life.

Natalie Smith Parra is a teacher, writer and activist who was diagnosed with inoperable lung cancer in 1996. Since then she has served as Artist in Residence for InsideOut Writers, teaching creative writing to incarcerated youth in Los Angeles. She is the recipient of several grants, awards and residencies for her writing, including Hedgebrook, Mesa Refuge and Norcroft, the Money for Women/Barbara Deming Memorial Fund grant and a Puffin grant. She is working on her second book of non-fiction. Natalie lives in Los Angeles, California. She has three children and two grandchildren.

Cancer Survivor
Sharon Burrell

I am forty-seven years old, happily married, with two absolutely precious children who are everything to me. I am an attorney, but have not practiced since I had my children. I have never smoked. I seem to have no other risk factors for lung cancer. But I got it.

Before I was diagnosed, I had chest pain for several years and a persistent cough for many months. My doctor kept telling me that I had a digestive disorder called GERD, a kind of acid reflux disease. I developed a slight feeling of not being able to take a deep breath. When I told my doctor that I couldn't breathe, she said, "But you *are* breathing, Sharon." I started to cry out of exasperation, and insisted on some testing.

A chest X-ray showed a 2.5 centimeter nodule. From there I had several CT scans. My pulmonologist thought I might have some weird infection. I was given antibiotics, more CT scans and finally a PET scan. Reviewing the results, the doctor, a very well respected surgeon, told me he didn't think I had cancer and sent me back to my pulmonologist. The pulmonologist offered me several options, one of which was a biopsy. I agreed and waited a long couple of weeks for the results. The first biopsy did not work. I had a second biopsy a week later. I called the surgeon for the results. He said, matter of factly, "Well, you do have a tumor."

That's how I found out I had Stage IA adenocarcinoma of the left lung, from the same surgeon who, a few weeks earlier, had told me he didn't think I had cancer. Apparently, my tumor did not "light up" on the PET scan the way cancer generally does. I have since learned that adenocarcinomas often do not show up well on PET scans. The surgeon scheduled me for surgery in two weeks. I spent those weeks getting my affairs in order and finding care for my family.

I mention all this because I want people to know that they must be aggressive and be their own advocate with cancer. When I first called for an appointment after my local doctor found the nodule on my lung, I was given their earliest appointment, which was over a month away. I thought that was totally unacceptable. I got in within a week by taking a cancellation that a very nice secretary let me have. But I had to be extremely assertive to get the appointment, the diagnosis and then to get the surgery.

I was offered chemotherapy because my tumor was so close in size to being 1B. Some studies have shown that chemotherapy can benefit stage 1B patients. After much thought, I decided not to have the treatment. It was a very difficult decision, but I felt that the chemotherapy might be too much for my body to handle and there didn't seem to be any studies that showed a significant benefit from the treatment for 1A patients.

I am told my prognosis is good, a five-year survival probability of 65% to 85%, depending on which doctor I ask or which study I read. I know that many people face a bleaker situation than mine, and my heart goes out to all of them. Cancer is a very frightening occurrence that totally changes your life. I'm hoping that, for me, as more time goes by, it gets a bit easier. My worst fear is not being here for my children. I have a considerable amount of pain, which, although I've been told is from the surgery (not that I really believe what any doctor says anymore), still scares me. I'm much better now than I was right after the surgery, but I still have some difficulty breathing and I feel a constant tightness in my throat and chest. I know that I have shown a lot of improvement; I don't cough much anymore for the first time in probably over a year. I should throw myself a party just for that!

Sharon is an attorney who has been married for twenty-four years. A mother of two, she lives in a small community outside Boston, Massachusetts.

Continued from page (89)

Choosing the Right Surgeon

Your case will fall into one of two broad, general categories. You have either a lung cancer that is curable and can be removed or eliminated, or one that can only be controlled, shrunk or improved.

In the case of a relatively small tumor with a high probability of malignancy or which was biopsied and found to be malignant, the tumor would be removed with surgery. Your regular physician would most likely refer you to a chest (*thoracic*) surgeon. The three most important factors to consider in deciding if this individual is right for you are his technical expertise, his medical background and his bedside manner. Also important in making this decision is the quality of the facility at which this physician performs surgery. If possible, obtain references from a few of his other patients or other healthcare providers who have worked with him in the past.

You will want someone who is skillful in conveying bad news and capable of dealing honestly yet tactfully with sensitive, life-threatening issues. In addition, he must be able to clearly explain the nature of your medical problem, the type of surgery that needs to be done, and any special issues that are important to your particular case using no technical jargon, so that you and your companion have a crystal clear understanding of the surgery, why it is needed and of any possible complications. You should be able to ask questions and receive clear, unhurried responses. You must not feel like you are just simply a number among many thousands of his patients. The following are warning signs that a surgeon you are considering may not be right for you:

- Lack of a reliable, positive recommendation or negative reports about the surgeon from other, reliable healthcare practitioners.

- A very busy office in which the atmosphere is so rushed that it appears you will not get the time to have your concerns addressed.

- He does not like to answer questions.

- He is evasive or his answers to your questions are fuzzy.

- The surgeon seems to recommend surgery without giving you time to consider other options or to get a second opinion.

- The surgeon gets annoyed when you indicate that you might wish to consider a second opinion.

Any of these issues should cause you to think about seeking your medical care elsewhere.

Continued on page (134)

My Journey with Lung Cancer

Doris Taylor

In January 2004, my daughter Suzanne was diagnosed with sciatica. She was treated for three months, but with no relief. Her doctor didn't order an MRI; he didn't think the insurance would pay for it. Four months later, when she appeared at the hospital emergency room for the third time for severe back pain, the test was finally done. The doctors discovered advanced lung cancer which had spread to the bones. Her doctor had her admitted to the hospital, but told us the cancer was too advanced to treat. She died three months later. Both her husband and I feel that if she had gotten the MRI earlier, she would have had a better chance for survival, or at least a longer time without the severe pain.

Not long after Sue's diagnosis, at an appointment of my own, I asked my doctor (not the same doctor as Sue's) to answer some of my concerns about lung cancer. I told her I felt fine, and had never smoked; however, I mentioned that my brother had died from lung cancer at age fifty-seven. She suggested that I have a chest X-ray.

I was shocked when the X-ray showed a tumor in my left lung. After a biopsy confirmed that it was cancer, my doctor scheduled me for a bone scan, a PET scan, an MRI and appointments with a surgeon and oncologist. I told them I was taking care of Sue and they could set it up, but I needed to be with my daughter for as long as she needed me. Unfortunately, she died the night after I saw my surgeon.

A month after all the tests were done, I had a left upper lobectomy. Luckily, there was no node involvement, so I didn't need chemotherapy. Everything happened so fast, I had no time to grieve for Sue. When I finally felt the pain of her loss, I was devastated. Just the mention of her name sent me off crying. Luckily for me, my church has a grief share program that I was able to attend; my church family and my friends helped me through this difficult time. I also attended a cancer support group at my hospital. It seemed to take months before I could hold back my tears when I spoke of her. Even now, I have difficult times.

Sue was my oldest child and my best friend. When I needed to "unload," she was always there to listen to me. I was there to listen to her. We confided in each other about everything, being sure not to interfere with each other's lives. She had a soft heart and a gentle manner. Sue and I were kindred spirits. She left behind two lovely children, a daughter, age sixteen and a son, age thirteen. They are doing as well as teens can do. They are very special, and we will always be there to support them. Her husband has also done pretty well, despite now having to manage everything by himself.

After my cancer, I did a family history. My brother died from lung cancer at age fifty-seven. My sister died from lung cancer the following year, at age sixty- three. My mother died from lung cancer at age sixty-four. My mother's two brothers also died from lung cancer. I am now enrolled in a genetics study at Wayne State University and another in Ohio. My two children are being tested. My daughter is a smoker, my son is not.

I am sixty-eight, and doing fine at this point. I volunteer at my church and at the hospital in the recovery room three days a week. I walk close to four miles a day. I have no shortness of breath or any other symptoms.

Because this disease may have a hereditary component, everyone who has lung cancer in their families should get checked often. Lung cancer is not always caused by smoking. I never smoked. More women than men get this very deadly cancer, which is curable if detected early. I hope that by sharing my experience, I can influence others to be alert and perhaps save lives.

The author, a retired nurse, celebrated her 50th wedding anniversary in 2006. A recovery room volunteer at the Kaiser Hospital, she resides in Sacramento, California.

It's a Great Life
if You Don't Weaken

Sharon Hindus

"In the attitude of silence the soul finds the path in a clearer light, and what is elusive and deceptive resolves itself into crystal clearness. Our life is a long and arduous quest after Truth."

—Mahatma Gandhi, Indian ascetic and nationalist leader (1869–1948)

The first thing many people say to me when they hear I have lung cancer is "How long did you smoke?" My answer: I smoked for five years, from 1973 to 1977, then quit cold turkey and never had another cigarette. Of course, I grew up in the 50's when everyone smoked, including my mom, dad, grandfather, aunts and uncles, my husband and in-laws. There was always a blue haze in the living room and a smoke film on the windshield of every car.

But I have read that five years after you've quit you are no longer in danger of getting lung cancer from smoking. I wonder how I got it. I've asked that question over and over, ever since my diagnosis of Stage IV advanced lung cancer, five years ago. I bet that they'll find out some day that extensive exposure to cigarette smoke during childhood makes us susceptible to lung cancer.

I was only fifty-one when I was diagnosed. I remember having a bad case of pneumonia in my early forties. I was given antibiotics and it went away. I also had a chest X-ray. If I had cancer then, the pneumonia would have blocked it out. The same thing happened just prior to my diagnosis in 2001. Then, I had a lot of pain and the building where I worked had an anthrax scare. My doctor grudgingly agreed to a chest X-ray "just to make me feel better." It showed a bad case of pneumonia, so I went to a pulmonary specialist. She said I looked too good to have pneumonia, and didn't think I needed a CT scan. But after two more weeks without a change in my condition she decided to do one. It took another week to read it at my small local hospital (the big hospitals in Boston read them within an hour). Then I got the call from my doctor: "It could be bad or really, really bad." She said. "You need to have a biopsy. We see a mass in your lung." The pneumonia had hidden the cancerous tumor in my right lung.

That's how I began my journey with this disease. My prognosis was not good; the surgeon who did my biopsy told my husband that I had maybe six to eight months, tops (his medical assistant calls me every year to see if I'm still here. I've been incredibly lucky: only 15% of lung cancer victims live over five years).

One day, I was a woman juggling a more than full-time job and the demands of being a wife and mother to two teenagers. The next day I was a cancer patient caught up in the whirlwind of technology and science trying to save my life. I became almost totally absorbed in fighting this disease.

I had been the sole breadwinner in the family since my husband's quadruple bypass heart surgery five years earlier, his severe hypertension and his later heart infection, which required a second open-heart surgery. Now I was the critically ill patient and he was my caregiver. Blind panic was a feeling I'd never experienced before. I cried a lot but that did nothing to change the fact that I had incurable lung cancer. I was like a two-year-old whose temper tantrums are being ignored. I tried to "numb out" but you know the "seeing your life flash before your eyes" bit? Well, I saw it for weeks. I saw it until I was sick of it! Finally I didn't want to mourn any more. I wanted to think about the future. That's when I knew I was going to live.

My major motivation to live was my husband and children: there was no way I would leave them without a fight. And it wasn't an issue of what I wanted, it's a core belief I hold, that life is about not giving up. I stopped feeling like I was being punished. In fact, I felt that in a way I had been given an opportunity to walk on a brand new path. Certainly, there were many times I felt totally overwhelmed by what was happening. But strength came to me the same way it always has: through meditation and prayer. When I'd done everything I could think of, I'd ask God for strength and peace of mind. Then, I could take another step forward, managing what I could and accepting what I couldn't.

By the end of my first year with lung cancer I had gone through menopause and survived a pulmonary embolism and two brain tumors. I lost all of my hair and most of my physical strength but my CT scan showed No Evidence of Disease (NED) in the lung and an MRI of my brain was clean.

My husband had promised me that the whole family would go to Hawaii to celebrate our victory through this first year. Hawaii had been on my wish list since I was a little girl. My grandfather had taken a trip there in 1917 and marveled at the black beaches and the volcanoes on the Big Island. We decided to island-hop between Kauai, Maui and Hawaii for almost three weeks beginning in late December.

Even if I couldn't hike, I could swim … well, glide around in the water. I got to be with my kids on their first scuba dive by using a raft to hold my tanks and a 20 foot air hose, which allowed me to use a minimal amount of energy. We dove into Molakini, a dormant volcano off the east coast of Maui. I felt nervous for only the first ten seconds of the dive, until I was sure that I'd have no trouble breathing. How incredible to have survived lung cancer and go diving in Hawaii, all in one year!

I believe we never would have done any of these things if I hadn't gotten cancer. Of course, the physical reality of the disease and its treatment has made me face my own mortality every day but, even during the initial shock and fear, I realized that I am now in a position to reflect upon these questions: What do I really believe? What will I make of my life? What do I really want? What a surprising and remarkable gift!

Two years ago, tests showed the tumor in my lung was growing and two more brain metastases were found, the third recurrence. They were successfully treated with Steriotactic Radio Surgery (SRS), the least invasive form of brain surgery. The idea of undergoing chemo overwhelmed me, but my doctors assured me there were many new drugs with which they were having some success, particularly with women who hadn't smoked. So there was a ray of hope.

My therapy plan was scheduled and I prepared my family and myself for this new battle. We'd been through a few operations— one to remove liquid from my lung that was making it difficult for me to breathe and two brain tumor removals. I had no idea what a siege this one was going to be. On the morning I was to go in for my third brain tumor procedure I had a horrific fall in a hotel room. The second I landed on that cold bathroom floor, I knew my entire universe had shifted. My surgical team was waiting in the emergency room when the EMTs brought me in. A vertebra in my lower back was crushed and I had broken three ribs. I couldn't do more than roll.

The next morning a very young German doctor visited me. He explained that the plan was to make a small incision in my back and thread a deflated balloon into the crushed vertebra, then inflate it and fill the gap with a kind of superglue. Once completed, he believed that I'd be able to stand up and walk. I said, "Great! Let's do it now!"

After four days I was finally able to stand up on my own, and two weeks before Christmas I was sent home. But I couldn't have the brain surgery until I could sit up for four to six hours. Every day my physical and occupational therapists put me through my paces while I was imprisoned in my dining room where they had installed a hospital bed, a wheelchair, a walker and a commode.

It was three months before my doctors felt I could endure the chemotherapy treatments. The good news (at least to me) was that I lost fifty pounds in those three months. My doctors, however, did not see this as a good thing, but rather a sign the cancer was becoming more aggressive and that I needed to get going on my treatment.

The next year was dedicated entirely to chemotherapy. We tried three different chemotherapy drugs before we found one that worked. I had my last chemotherapy session in December, 2005. My biggest problem since then has been ongoing battles with lung infections. This is part of what survivors have to deal with because of the effects of radiation on the bronchial tubes and lungs; it goes with the territory.

According to my last two CT scans, my cancer is hibernating but I'm still dealing with the challenge of having a chronic illness. The physical, psychological and economic realities of this disease make it difficult for survivors to remain a valued and productive part of society.

I'm out walking every day—slowly, but I have to keep getting out of the house. This week, for the first time in almost a year, I walked out to Pilot's Point, one half mile from my house.

The extent of my ability changes from week to week and this disease comes back to get me from time to time, but so far there are remedies. I can still write and talk on the phone. I volunteer as a phone buddy for the Lung Cancer Alliance and I've started writing about lung cancer and my experiences. The work answers one of those questions about the purpose of my life. It's amazing how important it is to talk to people who can truly empathize with you. It is a lifeline that I hope I can throw to people who are dealing with this life-threatening illness. I am not a lung cancer guru, but I want to be there to lend my experience and creativity to people living with this disease. I've discovered that I've gotten back even more than I've given.

So that's where I am right now. I'm doing it and while I do it I live and breathe. Like I say to my family, I'm not dying of cancer, I'm living with it. I'm reminded of a saying that my grandmother had for whenever anyone felt stressed out: it's a great life if you don't weaken.

The former Marketing Programs Manager with Digital Equipment Corporation's Corporate Information Systems Group, the author's expertise is being put to work through her writing, advocacy work to help others with life threatening diseases and as a volunteer phone buddy for the Lung Cancer Alliance. She lives with her husband, two teenage children and two dogs on the Taunton River in Somerset, Massachusetts.

Author's Note: I would like to dedicate this story to my lung cancer friends: Maureen, Judy, Laura, Doreen, Doug and Charlotte, Terrence and Rebecca, Carolyn, Linda (deceased) and Barry (deceased) and my family, friends and doctors who put up with me, took care of me and kept me going through all of this, even including the no-hair freak-out and the Decadron (a steroid better known as "bi-polar in a bottle.")

Life's Greatest Asset

Lori Monroe

Before September 2001, my life was ordinary. I was married, raising my two darling daughters and working full time as a nurse. Life was good, happy, uneventful, and wonderfully ordinary. Then I was diagnosed with Stage IV lung cancer, and my life as I had always known it ended.

It started with a hysterectomy, a common procedure for a 42 year-old woman like me. The pre-operative chest X-ray showed an infiltrate in one of the lobes of my lungs; probably pneumonia, nothing to worry about. The surgeon gave me intravenous antibiotics during the hospital stay to treat the pneumonia and I recovered from the surgery within days. I remember even feeling lucky to have six weeks off work.

Two weeks after surgery, I had another chest X-ray to follow up on the "pneumonia," but it hadn't cleared. My concern grew, yet I wasn't alarmed. I was healthy, I felt good, nobody thought too much of it. Then I had a CT scan. I can still remember the faces of the technicians as they watched the pictures come across the computer. The CT scan revealed an 8 centimeter mass in my left lower lobe and other nodules in my right upper lobe. We still didn't know what it was, but the tone had changed. My doctor suggested an immediate biopsy. I became more concerned, but the doctors were telling me that I was too young and healthy for it to be anything serious. I didn't have any risk factors for lung cancer and I didn't have any symptoms: I wasn't short of breath; I didn't have a cough or pain anywhere.

The pulmonologist called me the morning after the procedure and asked that I come in at lunchtime. I knew by the tone of his voice that he had bad news to deliver. A couple of hours later, I was sitting in his office, listening as he explained that, surprisingly, he had found a few cancer cells. My pre-cancer life had ended; my nightmare had begun.

Still, I focused on the words "few" and translated that to literally mean three. I thought we had caught the cancer early. I was fortunate to find the cancer early, and I silently kept telling myself over and over that I would be OK.

As a nurse, I knew the cardio-pulmonary surgeon well, so I called him on his cell phone. I tried to talk him into just taking me to surgery that evening, to take the cancer away. Even with my background I knew nothing about lung cancer. As a patient, I only knew I wanted it gone. He rightfully refused to agree to surgery that night. He said he wanted more tests and scans to make sure the cancer hadn't spread. I hadn't even thought of metastasis. I tried to remain confident that we had found the cancer early.

The next two days were full of every kind of scan imaginable, brain, bone, CTs, MRIs and lastly a PET scan. Confidently, we went ahead and scheduled the surgery for the third day, pending the scan reports. On the morning of the scheduled surgery, the surgeon came in and said to me, "I can't do your surgery." I didn't get it at first; I thought I was being 'bumped' for a more important case. But his face was somber. He said he had "looked at the PET scan and it didn't look good." I could feel the panic rise. I tried to talk him into going ahead with the surgery and then letting me do chemo or radiation afterwards for any remaining cancer. He kept saying, "I can't help you. Surgery won't help."

Finally, I heard him, and asked him where he thought he saw the cancer. I wasn't prepared for his answer. He replied slowly, "It's in your cervical spine, the lymph nodes around your neck, both clavicles, the lymph nodes around your aorta; the liver and both adrenal glands. The thoracic spine is consumed with it."

For the first time, I felt true panic, like all the air had been sucked from the room and I couldn't breathe. I felt numb. I remember thinking "I have children, I can't have cancer," as if being a mother somehow, made me immune.

After canceling my surgery, the surgeon made an appointment for me that same day with an oncologist I'd known for twenty years. I was confident she would be able to sort through this and would realize it was all a mistake. Instead, she told me I was in Stage IV and the cancer had metastasized throughout my body. She explained that while there were a few chemo agents for lung cancer, they weren't very effective. She added that we could look into some clinical trials. However, based on what she could see, she thought our real decision should be if we even wanted to start treatments. She coolly spoke of "quality of life," a term I quickly came to despise. I thought my quality of life should be to live. She said that at this time, I could take care of and enjoy my family, but if I started treatments I would become sicker more quickly, with the end result being the same. Stonily, she gave me a prognosis of six to ten months with treatment, six to eight months without. I was devastated. I never went back to see her again.

I felt as though my life was unraveling. All the pieces were still there, however nothing was cohesive anymore. I've worked in critical care all my life and was able to make split-second life-saving decisions, and now I couldn't decide what to eat for breakfast. The medical world, where I had spent half my life, became intimidating overnight. Nothing felt familiar; the sounds of the hospital were too loud, the lights too bright and harsh. It was as foreign as the cancer residing within me. My confidence in all I knew was gone.

The next few days I tried to re-group, to sort through what I had been told and what I knew. I had major decisions to make without the ability or knowledge to make them. I went for a second opinion at Vanderbilt University Medical Center in Nashville, Tennessee. It was there that I met Dr. Mathew Ninan, the first doctor to allow me any hope. A thoracic surgeon, he told me he didn't believe that I had as much tumor burden as I had first been told, but he was very concerned about the right lung. He believed, correctly, that the PET scan readings were inaccurate. I was ecstatic. Finally, someone realized this was all a mistake.

My joy was short-lived. During a surgery to check the nodules on my right lung Dr. Ninan found cancer. It had been around two weeks from my first diagnosis. I was still Stage IV, and at first he said he would not be able to help me either. That was possibly my lowest day. I felt I had gone full circle and arrived at the same prognosis. There was nothing left to do. I spent that day trying to accept that my time was limited. I clearly remember my conversations with my best friend Annette and with my husband. We spoke of the past, of memories, of what I wanted for my children's future. Annette promised to always be in my children's lives, David promised to never give up on life. We laughed, we cried, we mourned and in the end we were silent together. For the first time I began to accept what was happening.

Late that same night, Dr. Ninan called me and changed everything. He told me he had been thinking about my case, and if I still wanted him to do my surgery, he would do it. He was giving me back hope. He told me he didn't know if it would change my prognosis, but he didn't know that it wouldn't either. I agreed to his offer immediately; what did I have to lose? One week later, I had a second surgery to remove the largest tumor.

Over the next couple of weeks, as I recovered from the surgeries, I found the greatest oncologist, Dr. David Carbone. He straight away explained that although I was Stage IV and incurable, that in no way meant I was untreatable. His plan was simple—prevent metastasis for the next twenty years! His theory is to treat cancer as a chronic illness, something that leaves room for hope. I soon came to realize the difference between good doctors and great physicians. Great physicians—and there are truly very few of them—not only allow you to maintain hope, they will loan you theirs when you are running low.

Two months after the surgeries, I began a clinical trial of chemotherapy that lasted most of the next year. I found that some of the most difficult days were yet to come, both physically and emotionally. I came to hate the word "cancer". I had difficulty even walking through the doors of the cancer clinic to receive treatment. Some days it would literally take me several attempts just to walk in. I wasn't afraid of the treatments or the pain; it was the knowledge that I belonged there, that I had cancer.

The hardest part of my life with cancer has been facing it with my daughters. I felt as though I had somehow let them down. I knew I wasn't ready to let them go; they weren't ready, they were too young. I didn't know how much or what to tell them about my illness. They were ten and thirteen at the time; just beginning their teenage years, a time when they needed me the most. It broke my heart to feel that I would be responsible for the harshest pain they would ever experience, yet I wouldn't be there to comfort them in my death. I feared what they would have to witness and endure, knowing how ugly and cruel cancer can be. As a mother, I had promised to always be there for them, to teach them life-lessons, to prepare them for their future. Now, I would betray their precious trust. Even before cancer, I felt I was born to become their mother; they are the focus and purpose of my life. Now cancer threatened to steal this joy from me.

Since my journey first began, I have had many ups and downs. In December 2002, after the first two surgeries and the year of chemo, I had another lung surgery. And my marriage failed. I don't believe cancer was the reason for my divorce. I think cancer, or any major stress, works to magnify what is already there. If it is good, it only gets better, if it is shaky, it crumbles. My marriage crumbled.

After the third surgery, I was cancer-free for almost eighteen months. But in April 2004 another lesion was found in the upper lobe of my left lung. After careful and thoughtful consideration, we decided on another lung surgery to remove the new tumor. I expected to be able to handle a recurrence with greater confidence, but it was not any easier; if anything, it was harder. At the very least, it was different. I didn't feel the same panicked need to have it removed within the hour. I had the knowledge that comes with understanding what a recurrence signifies. The cancer resides within my body, waiting to interrupt life at any given time, threatening my life, shattering my world, stealing my ability to make plans past three months.

In December 2005, I had another recurrence, this time in the right lung's upper lobe. Once again, my great surgeon, Mathew Ninan, successfully removed it. That was my fifth lung surgery. All together, he has removed over half my lung tissue, yet I still feel healthy. I can still breathe, I still work as a nurse, I still have life and most importantly, I am still my daughters' mother. They are now fifteen and eighteen and over the past five years we have shared in some brilliant memories, faced our fears, lived multiple life lessons and enjoyed precious time together.

While I will never be one of those survivors who claim that cancer is the best thing that ever happened to them, it has in many ways enlightened me. It has given me a greater appreciation and love for my family and friends around me: the knowledge that every day, every moment is precious; that our greatest asset is simply time; that while I cannot control what happens to me, I can control how I react to it. While I may die from cancer, it can never, never defeat me.

Lori Monroe was diagnosed at age 42 with Stage IV non-small cell lung cancer. She has two beautiful teenage daughters, Alyson and Emily, who are her inspiration and who have given her courage to fight her disease. Emily's story also appears in this book. An emergency room registered nurse, Lori is a patient advocate for The National Cancer Institute's Lung Specialized Programs of Research Excellence (SPORES), a multi-million dollar grant program that funds institutions undertaking specialized research into lung cancer. She is also a patient representative with National Cancer Institutes, Eastern Cooperative Oncology Group (ECOG), an association of doctors and researchers who collaborate to conduct clinical cancer trials. Lori has been featured in *The Wall Street Journal* and has worked with the Lance Armstrong Foundation.

Part IV

RECONNECTING

Sooner or later we must realize there is no station, no one place to arrive at once and for all. The true joy of life is the trip.

—*Robert J. Hastings*

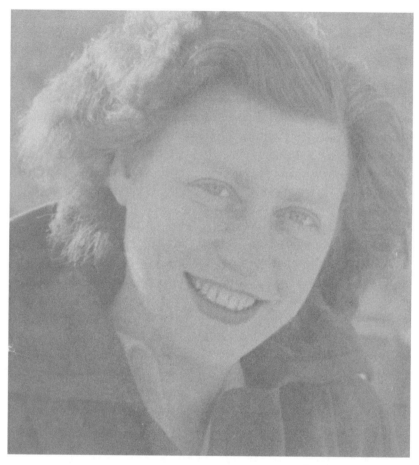

Elisabeth Buchhalter Segal, page 45

Now I Understand
Barbara Terrell

I get it. No, I *really* get it. It took almost three years and a bout of breast cancer, but I now understand my mother-in-law, Julie.

I always thought that my husband, Eric, had married the exact opposite of his mother. Julie raised two children and never sat still. Her days were filled with charitable committee meetings, church activities, and Jazzercise; my days were filled with work meetings, church on Saturday nights and dog walks. Julie kept her petite figure by eating nothing but fruits and vegetables and low-fat foods; I believe eating pizza every day covers all the food groups. She raised her kids to eat healthy and stay active; I feed her son Lucky Charms for breakfast. She dressed like she could grace the cover of a fashion magazine, accessorizing with imaginative southwestern jewelry or scarves; I live in blue jeans and turtlenecks and have been known to show up at work with no earrings and two different colored socks. Yup, we were as different as night and day.

Eric and I had been married for about a year and had just spent the holidays with Julie and Bob, Eric's dad. Julie was vibrant and healthy, but had a touch of laryngitis, which she laughed off as being due to too much talking. She'd been hoarse for a month, and after a day of skiing decided she should probably go to the doctor. Then came her phone call. I instantly knew something was wrong. When I answered the phone there was no small talk, Julie wanted to talk to Eric right away. The doctor had taken a chest X-ray and made a grim discovery. She had lung cancer. Eric held the phone to his chest and silently cried.

Shocked and wanting to be involved as much as possible, Eric and I drove from Denver to Santa Fe and went to see the doctor with Julie and Bob. I felt like an outsider at the oncologist's office—my family dies of heart attacks and strokes. How does one handle cancer? When the doctor told us that the cancer was inoperable and had been found outside of her lungs, Bob, Julie, and Eric knew what that meant. Julie's sister had died of lung cancer a few years earlier.

From that day, I never heard Julie complain about having lung cancer. (She did complain about wearing a wig that made her head itch, and about having so many doctor appointments.) When her chemo schedule permitted, she kept going to her committee meetings and when she was feeling strong enough, Jazzercise. She loved being around people and keeping busy. She rarely varied her routine. Julie stayed up all hours of the night, as if she had to squeeze thirty hours into every twenty-four. Eric and I were puzzled. We wanted Julie to spend more time with her grandchildren and frankly, with us. Instead, Julie planned the yearly garage sale fundraiser for her pet charity, American Association of University Women. We tried to visit her once a month, but it always seemed like she was busy; I felt as if we were interrupting her schedule. But she always made sure her plans never interfered with our visits.

Julie was very resilient. She made it through chemotherapy. She made it through radiation treatments when the cancer went to her brain. Julie then volunteered to take part in a clinical trial for the new drug Iressa, which gave her six months of Indian summer: remission. Then, two and a half years after her initial diagnosis, the cancer was back with a vengeance. Bob was devastated when he had to call hospice.

Eric and I spent two weeks with Julie while she was under hospice care at home. There were times when she wasn't lucid. Other times, she was the old Julie, trying to organize and plan. Julie was worried she was putting everyone out and, of all things, that she had bad breath. It was during one of her lucid times that she insisted Eric and I take a few days and go on a long-planned vacation. I thought she was nuts but she insisted. Not wanting to upset her, we tearfully said what we believed would be our last good-byes and left for two days. We were nervous wrecks, calling and checking on her several times a day, racked with guilt, afraid we wouldn't be there when she and Bob needed us.

During our return to Santa Fe, Julie had slipped into a coma. We were told the end was near. I was sitting with her, holding her hand, telling her about the Indian ruins we'd visited and how we wished she had been with us. Her breathing became erratic. I ran and got Bob, Eric, and Julie's sister, Francie. We were gathered around her, touching her and telling her how much we loved her when Julie took a rasping breath and was gone.

I always wondered why Julie was so determined to maintain her schedule and to make sure that everyone maintained theirs. In a way, I felt like we'd been gypped out of spending more time with her. Try as I might, I couldn't understand it.

Fast forward three years. Eric and I were sitting in a $2 movie theater watching the Johnny Depp movie *Finding Neverland*. During one scene near the end of the movie, the mother insists that her kids go to a play, even though she was dying. Throughout the movie, she tried to make sure that everything was as routine as possible for her kids, trying to shield them from her suffering. Her death scene so reminded Eric and me of Julie's death that we both started to cry uncontrollably. And then, a light bulb dimly flickered to life in my mind, a hint of a thought.

A few months later, I had my own shocking phone call. I was diagnosed with DCIS, ductal carcinoma in situ, an early stage of breast cancer. I had bilateral lumpectomies and four lymph nodes removed, followed by five weeks of radiation treatments. While my prognosis is totally positive, I discovered that cancer is all-consuming. Cancer swallowed my life, and then spit it out and I'm still trying to clean up the mess.

During my recovery, I was fanatical in proving to myself that I wasn't any different, that I could still handle my usual routine. Three days after my surgery, I cleaned out the refrigerator. Six days after surgery, I went on a two mile hike. The next day, I went on an annual elk hunt with my father and hiked five miles before driving four hours back to Denver. (I don't carry a gun; I take scenery photographs.) I wasn't going to let a little thing like breast cancer make me cancel a 21-year family tradition!

Every day I worked full-time. Every day I did physical therapy so I could raise my arm. (I had lymphedema, which made it difficult for me to use my left arm.) Although it was embarrassing to be caught by co-workers standing in the bathroom looking like the Statue of Liberty trying to stretch out my arm, I kept telling myself I'd be back to normal soon, to hang in there, to keep a positive attitude.

Normalcy: that was what I craved. I wanted to be able to exercise like I used to. I wanted to be able to close my car door with my left arm. I wanted my husband to give me a chest massage because I'm sexy, not because he needed to break up my scar tissue. I didn't want to be labeled a breast cancer survivor, but just a normal person doing normal everyday things. Then, the dim light bulb in my brain that had flickered on at the movies started to shine at 100 watts. Normalcy: that was exactly what Julie had coveted. She just wanted to be a normal person, not someone dying from lung cancer. Suddenly, Julie's behavior made perfect sense.

I guess we weren't so different after all.

Prompted to start writing non-fiction by a bout with breast cancer, Barbara has been giving corporate presentations since 1987. Her goal is to help others realize that they can make it through challenging times with humor. She lives in a suburb of Denver with her computer guru husband, a shy yet neurotic German Shepard, and a cat she calls "the evil one."

Continued from page (107)

Getting a Second Opinion

In my opinion, the best practice is to get a second opinion regarding proposed lung surgery. If the surgeon appears to present some of the danger signs mentioned in the preceding paragraph, a second opinion is mandatory. If he suggests in any way that your case is unusual or if you are at a particularly high risk because of an unusual medical situation, you need a second opinion. If there is a question whether the abnormality on the chest X-ray or CT scan is malignant or whether you need surgery, you need a second opinion. If you are unsure of how to proceed or are especially worried about the outcome of the surgery, get a second opinion.

You are not required to use the services of the chest surgeon who gives you the second opinion. Many second opinion specialists aggressively seek to convince you to allow them to perform the surgery by making negative remarks about the first surgeon. It may also seem easier to stick with the second surgeon. However, if the second opinion gives you the same analysis and treatment plan as the first and your initial surgeon satisfied all of your criteria, I recommend sticking with the first surgeon, especially if he is closer to where you live. If the surgeon giving the second opinion says something radically different from the first and you believe it to be the best course of action, or if your case requires technology or treatment that can only be had where the second surgeon practices, that is where you should have your surgery. You also have the option of getting a third opinion if the first two opinions are contradictory or very different. Surgery for lung cancer is not usually a medical emergency and taking a few weeks to get additional opinions on your medical situation can be worthwhile.

Continued on page (140)

Always Treasure Today
Michael Steven Edwards

To hear a doctor say you only have a few months to live must sound unbelievable to anyone. It was no different for my father. After a yearly physical followed by some additional tests, his doctors told him he had lung cancer and only six to eighteen months to live. He had been a heavy smoker most of his adult life but had successfully quit ten years before. His doctors told him the cancer was not a direct result of smoking.

I learned about Dad's diagnosis when he unexpectedly came to my office. I usually saw my family only on the major holidays, such as Christmas or Thanksgiving. Even then, I kept my visits as brief as I could manage, always using the excuse that I had some important engagement to keep. The truth was, I couldn't stand the tension I felt being around them, and later on, I couldn't be away from alcohol for more than a .few hours without beginning to shake and sweat. "The results say I might have cancer," he told me that day, "but they're still running tests." I could see the fear in his eyes. A vulnerability that I had never seen in him before stirred my heart. It was more than my usual feelings of overwhelming guilt and rejection. This was something very different. It evoked in me feelings of worry and concern for him that I didn't know I had. I felt a need to be close to him and what I had always assumed had been my anger and hatred towards him began to melt. I did not want him to die with us still at odds and I wanted to make sure he knew that, deep down, I loved him.

I made an effort to spend time doing yard work and other chores at his house on my free days. I had to show him I cared. My drinking was no secret and it disappointed him, but I went out there anyway. He clung to the hope that he would be cured or at least have the disease arrested so he could relax and enjoy all of the things he had saved up for all his life. I learned from this whole experience that you'd better live your life in a reasonably happy way today. The "magic day" you wait for, to let yourself loose to enjoy all of those things for which you worked so long, may never come.

Dad ended up living for just over four years from the day he told me of his diagnosis and he was able to see many remarkable things. I think the proudest day of his life was the day of my sister's wedding. It was a huge affair and he didn't nickel and dime it. I was asked to usher at the wedding two months before, a gesture that utterly broke my heart. The wedding was to take place in Santa Fe, New Mexico. It was to be a week-long event with rehearsals and dinners and entertaining, with lots of people to meet. This meant I would be out of my element and not in control of my time, an alcoholic's worst nightmare.

My alcoholism had progressed to daily drinking. It was a seven-day-a-week physical addiction over which I had no control and of which I was terribly ashamed. There was no way I could participate in the rehearsals and meet everyone without somehow embarrassing my family. Little did I know that a huge change in my life, by which God would enable me to get sober, would happen within weeks. It happened, and I have remained sober ever since. God works in ways that are indeed mysterious, marvelous and magnificent. I was able to be the most awkward, nervous usher you have ever seen, but I was so glad to be a part of it all.

The wedding was beautiful. Dad was asked to make a speech at the reception. He was extremely nervous. Of course he left his notes at the hotel. The truth is, he had given speeches and talks in front of some of the most powerful executives and government officials in the country. But this was the one that mattered. I told him funny stories and got him laughing and he pulled it off beautifully.

Dad went through many changes as the cancer spread. He was able to fight it with chemotherapy in the early days. I was so proud of him when he came to the country club for Thanksgiving dinner. He'd lost his hair but he made it. In my opinion, that would be difficult for anyone, but especially for someone as self-conscious as Dad.

Later, the cancer spread to his brain and he began radiation treatment. Compared to a year of chemotherapy, the side effects from these treatments were less severe. Still, his breathing was worsening, and we had to be very careful to shield him from any type of infection. He needed oxygen when he was at home. At times, Dad would have his breathing treatments and then be up and running around, shopping, seeming happy, as if he were perfectly healthy. Other times he was very difficult to deal with and in a terrible mood, or just sick and out of it.

He was hospitalized a few times during his fight with cancer, usually for an infection and once, in the third year, for a heart attack. Then came the day his blood pressure fell to almost nothing. It would not maintain its normal range, and after being rushed by ambulance to the emergency room, he was kept for observation.

I was able to devote most of my time to caring for him. I was at the hospital every night the first week. One night, we had a talk that laid everything on the table. There were no more secrets after that and he told me he was proud of me. When I told him I was proud of him, he asked me why. He never realized how lucky I felt, having such an accomplished dad. He told me he wished he could have done something to have changed or helped me early on. I told him the truth was that I would have turned out the way I did no matter what family raised me. I honestly believe that. Then he changed the subject, so we didn't get too emotional.

His cancer spread to his bones through his blood stream, and his doctor wanted to do a spinal tap, to find out if it had progressed to his spine. The following day, I was with him when he was told the results: he was now beyond the possibility of successful treatment. I saw the look of a condemned man in his eyes. He really hadn't accepted the possibility of death until then. I was glad I was there and that he wasn't alone.

My parents lived in a very exclusive, gated golf course community and Dad's doctor was a neighbor. Dad tried to make small talk with him about improvements in the neighborhood; I could sense the doctor keeping my dad at arms length. I felt so sorry for Dad right then. He was trying to have a dignified conversation with one of his equals, all the while feeling unequal because of his prognosis.

I wanted to jump inside him and scream out how damn dignified he should feel for all of the great things he had accomplished! He didn't need to feel bad about dying; he should have felt great about how he had lived his life! But he didn't. He had lost perspective on what mattered and what didn't. It enraged me. He seemed like a little kid just trying to make conversation to ease his fears of the unknown. He was terrified of dying, he was in a situation beyond his control and he knew it. And I knew there was nothing I could do to fix it.

Dad was never a religious person but he did start watching religious services and shows on television at the hospital. I was able to share with him the miracles that had led to and followed my getting sober. I think this had a profound effect on him, or it at least allowed him to see the huge change that had come over me. The same minister who performed my sister's wedding shared something with Dad about the Apostles Creed that was very significant to him, but only they knew what that was.

Now it was time to rest, but first we had to move him home. He was in intense pain by this time, as the cancer had begun to close his airway. There was no treatment other than radiation, which would keep his airway open only for a few more weeks. But he wanted to go home: my sister would be bringing her new baby home in six days, the day after Christmas. I helped transport him to and from the hospital on the Med Bus each day for radiation though the entire process. It was unbearable for him, and I thought it did more harm than good. But he wanted to make it long enough to see the baby. Throughout all of this, he and I became closer and closer, with him now dependent on me. He died Christmas Day. Although he hadn't lived to see his grandchild, I know that Dad's determination to see him kept him alive a little longer. So in this sadness I try to hold onto the memory of our treasured moments together. Those moments were far too few, but the love we both felt during that time will last forever.

Michael Edwards is a new writer from Oklahoma City, Oklahoma. At age forty-three he began writing poetry and has recently begun to write short stories. He divides his time between helping people less fortunate than himself and writing. Having lived an interesting life fraught with difficulties, he tries to live each day as if it was the only one that existed.

Continued from page (134)

Choosing an Oncologist

What if your tumor cannot be removed surgically because of its location or because it has *metastasized*, spread outside the original site of the cancer? You will probably be referred to a medical oncologist, who generally directs the care of a lung cancer patient facing this type of situation. This specialist determines and administers the medical treatment used to shrink or eliminate the tumor and conducts periodic diagnostic testing to determine your body's response to the therapy and the course of the illness. In addition, she will refer you to other specialists, such as the radiation oncologist, to treat certain aspects of your illness when necessary.

In selecting the best oncologist for you, use the criteria previously mentioned for picking any physician involved in your medical care. In addition, keep in mind that chemotherapy treatments can be physically taxing and you need to conserve your limited strength to fight your illness. Therefore, you should avoid long commutes to your chemotherapy sessions and, if at all possible, find a local facility. There are many well qualified medical oncologists with excellent bedside manners who practice in small to mid-sized communities and hospitals. It is not necessary to get an extended period of chemotherapy care at a large institution that is far away from home. Besides, if you need emergency assistance, it is almost impossible to get back quickly to a distant major medical center for care. You may end up in the local emergency room without the medical records available on your case, and a new group of physicians must start your treatment from scratch.

Continued on page (184)

Holding the Gray of Winter
Molly Jo Rose

It was winter when my mother first told me she had lung cancer. I was alone in my apartment in downtown Grand Rapids. Her voice came over the phone like a cold wind. All I could do was think about the snow. It somehow threatened to come in and cover me in goose bumps. It suggested that the color of fall would never return.

The truth of living in Michigan is that eventually, all things will turn cold and fade into one hundred shades of gray. There is one short minute in fall when the weathermen speak of percentages of color, and Michiganders take leisurely drives up North for a color tour. We take in all we can, like bears storing fat for hibernation, so that the gray of winter will not win. Sometimes spring does not come until late April, and during those winter months you can't help but start to mistrust the return of spring.

There was still some orange in the trees outside my window as my mother and I sat in silence across the phone line, she not knowing what to say next, I not wanting to hear what I had just heard. I waited for her to speak.

"I didn't want to tell you this way," my mother said. "But it turns out I have lung cancer." My mother's voice, the way she told me, the way she had said it with that resignation, would become too familiar, as if she deserved this slow death from the beginning.

I spent a good portion of the next three weeks learning everything I could about the disease. "Did you know," I once told her across the phone lines, "that there has always been cancer. They knew what it was, like, five thousand years ago." I knew she was not interested in talking about it, and she would do just about anything to get off the phone with me.

"Okay," my mom interrupted. "That's enough. I really don't want to hear this."

"You don't want to hear any more?" I looked down at the words staring back at me from the page of notes. I was dying to tell her what the Edwin Smith Papyrus predicted. It had only been a few weeks, but I had hardened in that way only career academics and doctors are capable of. Knowledge is its own avoidance drug. We always understand more than everyone else does. Knowledge is our shield from reality.

December came, and we had not felt the worst of the snow or the cancer. My mother and I sat at a booth in a restaurant with our menus splayed out across the table and our coats still on to keep in the warmth. Still trying to hide, I said, "Did you know cancer was named after the crab because the blood vessels surrounding the malignant tumors reminded Hippocrates of a crab?" My mom mostly ignored me and was obviously relieved when the waitress asked what we would like.

I knew what she would order—a vegetarian wrap called the No Meat This Time, which she ordered so often that I began calling it the *No Meat This Time Every Time*. But before she could order it, and before I could make my joke, an old friend of my mother's stopped to say hello. My mother had just begun her treatment and still looked well. She still had a full head of hair, and the color of her skin was still human and real looking, not yet that plastic hue of cheaply made dolls. Even a Michigan winter had more color than a person on cancer treatments.

"Oh, Dianne." The words oozed from his mouth like slushy water.

I could tell he knew my mom was sick before he said a word because his head was cocked just so, falling nearly to his shoulder as if it might roll right off. Mom seemed to know what was coming, too. Her eyes were dancing like they could hardly get rid of the moment fast enough. I slowed down my heartbeat, trying to balance hers out. It had always been this way between us. My therapist used to tell me, *you two work through osmosis.*

"Oh, Dianne," Ted said, probably meaning for it to sound right, to sound convincing and kind and unassuming. He offered it like a friendly handshake, but it came at her like a fist, plowing into my mother like a ruthless uppercut. I knew she felt it this way because I felt it this way. He asked with that cock of the head that would become disgustingly familiar and that sympathetic dip of the shoulders, "Did you smoke?"

How I will grow to hate those damning words coming from doctors and neighbors, all trying to show concern. Again and again reminding my mother of her accountability, of how much she was to blame for this.

In the dark crevices of a high shelf in my mother's closet, I found a leather photo album. Pasted inside were pictures of my teenage mother lounging around a lake with others her age. In these photos, my mother's brown eyes are resilient and hard, like Sophia Loren's in the poster of her coming off the beach that my father has hanging in his workshop.

My dad told me about this poster one evening as I watched him rattle through his enormous red toolbox. He searched for a bolt as I stared at the hard, confident image of Sophia Loren plastered across the unfinished wall of his workshop. It was the first time I realized my dad did not see my mother for who she'd become. On his knees, bent over the toolbox, he motioned up to the larger-than-life body whose eyes seared through the thin poster. "Your mother looks like her," he said.

In these album photos, cancer has not caught up with her. I mentally cataloged each photograph before asking her when these were taken, worried that she would take the book from me.

With a smile, she pulled the book into her lap. "I was at Houghton Lake," she told me, gently flipping through the yellowed pages. "I used to go there every year with a group of my friends." I know that pristine Northern Michigan lake with the black silhouettes of tall pines trees crowning it, taller than the ones crowding our backyard.

"How old were you?" I asked.

"Well," she said as she glanced through a few more pages before settling on a collection of photos on one page. In each photo, she was smoking. "I was seventeen in that one." She fingered the photo, and I turned the album toward me. The photographs were the die-cut kind, with scalloped edges and the month and year appear on each of the edges. The year, 1958, suggested my mother was fourteen. "No," I said. "You were fourteen."

She rotated the album in her direction.

"Hmm," she said, and then had to agree, "fourteen."

The truth of cancer, like the truth of a Michigan winter, is that you start to think it will never go away. It infiltrates you to the bone, wrestles its way in and chills you, an icy layer forming on all your parts just to survive. You hope for recovery like you hope for spring, but there's a part of you that cannot depend on it.

Every Thursday, a group of my mother's women friends came to her home and prayed with her. They recited the rosary and at every tenth Hail Mary, I heard my mother's voice reciting the mantra, "Jesus Christ, we want to be well." Her voice was thick with fear, and I did not stop shivering until their singing floated up the stairwell to me from the first floor where they were circled around a table with a statue of the Virgin Mary in the center. That singing meant they would leave soon. I let it warm me. Then I returned to my studies that filled my brain like a calming white-out of snow.

We forge our memories like hot irons against coal. We press against images and snippets of information like a white-hot light, weeding out the middle parts of conversation and remembering only the first and the last words. *I have something to tell you … it might be cancer.* That your mother will die is never obvious enough. It cannot be. It is the memory we cannot remember, the idea we cannot digest, the one we cannot press into the hard coal of memory with the hardest of hammers. That your mother will die means you will die. There is nothing lost in the translation of it.

The oblong room where my mother lay flat on her back, her tattoo exposed and ready, was cream-colored from ceiling to wall to machine to floor. Doctor Kane's white coat was suddenly glaring. "Please," he asked my mother, "Lay still, Dianne." As if she could possibly move in that state of paralyzing fear. It was the first day of therapy, and her knuckles gripped the sides of the cream cushioned table until they were as white as Doctor Kane's coat. My dentist had nicknamed me "White Knuckles" and I could see from whom I had inherited that propensity. I feared what else we might have in common.

"Just lie still and everything will be fine." The doctor's voice was like sugar, like a song. "You can leave the room now," he told me, and I waited for my mom to okay it. Her head jerked in an imitation of a nod. I waited for her to override the doctor's orders, but he shooed me out. I left her there alone with him.

It was only twenty minutes and then she was returned to me. Her voice was cracking in the fits of that familiar cough, one I had been hearing for years without alarm. It echoed down the tiled corridor like a dislodged metronome, ticking, reminding, this is the way the tune is played, this is your part and your responsibility. Walk down the hallway. Meet her. Hold her hand. Make everything okay. You are responsible for everything.

On a cellular level, the race is between metastasis and the combined treatment of radiation and chemotherapy. Metastasis is the spread of cancerous cells to remote parts of the body away from the primary tumor. The cancerous cells are capable of moving quickly and spontaneously. As they rush away from the primary growth, they look for a new organ where they can establish a new tumorous colony. Some cancer cells will invade a lymphatic vessel and travel in the lymph until they reach a lymphatic gland and deposit themselves there.

This is what happened to my mother. The primary growth was in her left lung. Then the quickly dividing cancer cells raced down to her lymph nodes, where they remain tightly entrenched. It is a race against metastasis, and my mother did not win. But neither has the metastasis. At this point, they are at a standstill. Every month, my mom goes in to confirm that the small growth remains its diminutive size. It waits and she waits, always fearful of its spontaneous movement returning, always aware that she is in a quiet race against death and the cancer cells attacking her lung are ultra-marathoners.

It is five years since her diagnosis, since we learned, with the swing of a hammer into our brains, that cancer had found us and would be staying for the long haul. I think sometimes, especially while shopping for wigs that could never replace the authenticity of my mother's salt-and-pepper hair, that we are swimming through something too thick, a sludge of gray stew that yanks at our feet and pulls us into darker waters that threaten to ice over and keep us trapped underneath. But I have too much of my father in me, a man who cannot see how much space has come between now and when my mother looked like a forties movie siren. I can be delightfully oblivious when necessary and escape the cancer by intervals, squirreling myself away to the outdoors, where the bleeding hearts have returned. These beautiful plants help us remember blood in a new way, not coming out from my mother's mouth, but spilling down from a pink, heart-shaped flower in the spring, which has finally returned.

I left my large windowed home on Crescent Street to move in with my parents, to always be there, just in case. Outside the windows of their home is a perennial garden, one my mom prunes and digs at as soon as the ground is soft enough. I see her smiling and squinting in the sunlight, her floral-gloved hand forming a visor over her eyes. I walk out the door and down the steps of the porch, which are saddled with sad clumps of melting snow. They will not survive past the warming sunlight of day.

My mother looks well again. Her hair is sprouting like the little shoots in the ground, eager and comely in its way, and she is soft again, like the picture in the photo album, forgetful of all the comments and the fears that have weighted her down, weighted us all down, for what seems like a lifetime.

"You know," I tell her, handing her a veggie sandwich; just the way she likes it. "You know it's not your fault. People smoke all the time and don't get sick. Your dad did. Lots of people do." It is a better kind of information to share with her, but I am only just learning that.

She shrugs, her shoulders so light they could float right off. "I know. I've figured that out already." And then she looks at me with those eyes, those searing eyes that tell me *I'm about to tell you something important, so pay attention.* "It can be offered up and made a prayer," my mom says. "Even those things we bring upon ourselves."

There's that prayer again. That miracle drug, more powerful than the radiation, chemotherapy, knowledge in books. She trusts it, so I do, too.

We work through osmosis, holding the gray of winter in our hands, but we're not responsible for it. We can pray over it, make it a friend or refuse it and let it beat against the window, perspire there, and suck away all the color. We choose to hold it fast. Spread it like seeds in the soil of our blood. We wait through the winter for spring to come and make the seeds into something good. Did she smoke? Yes, she did. And it hasn't killed us yet.

After her mother survived lung cancer, Molly Jo Rose returned to school to finish her Bachelor's Degree and is now working on her second Master's Degree in Creative Writing at Western Michigan University. She derives great inspiration from the cold and dark of Michigan winters.

Rediscovering Daddy
Susan Long

Jack of Diamonds, Jack of Diamonds
I've known you from old.
You've robbed my poor pockets
Of silver and gold.

Daddy loved to drive. He'd hop up on U.S. 119 along the Elk River between Clendenin and Charleston, West Virginia and we'd fly down the two-lane road, windows open, with him singing *Jack O' Diamonds*. "Why are you such a horrible singer, Daddy?" I'd ask. He would laugh, and then he'd sing even louder as he put the pedal to the metal.

I was only about ten years old then. I recall my daddy years later, sitting in his rocking chair with his head hung over from exhaustion and pain. Even then, he still wanted to go in the car. Only those times, I drove.

Driving together one of those times, as we merged onto the interstate, he looked over at me.

"Do you like to drive?" he asked.

"I love to drive," I lied.

"I always thought I should have been a truck driver," he said. "Could've driven all over the country and seen a lot."

To change the subject, I asked, "Will you sing *Jack O' Diamonds* for me?"

That's just one of many memories I have of my daddy. I'm fifty-three years old now, and my question reflected the instinctive knowledge that what makes our hearts sing at ten probably has the same effect on us when we're adults. But maturity has also taught me that when *my* heart sings, I need to return the gift.

The six-month period which began with his diagnosis of lung cancer in May, 2005, and ended when he died on November 22, 2005, became a lifetime—a shortened lifetime by normal standards, but one filled with moment after moment, hour after hour, day after day of rediscovering my daddy. During the Meso Lifetime, as I now refer to it, there were no days, no weeks, no seasons. Time seemed suspended. But the clock kept ticking.

My parents divorced when I was twelve and my two sisters and I moved away from West Virginia with my mom when I was fourteen. Over the years, I'd see my father maybe once a year, sometimes every other year. In some ways our relationship was frozen in time, which I guess is why I still call him Daddy.

Daddy remarried shortly after he and my mom divorced, and he had another daughter. He wasn't a great communicator; we didn't talk much between our infrequent visits and I always waited for him to make the first move. He didn't, but my stepmother, Dee, did. Our visits were always enjoyable, but I didn't mind when they ended. But then one day, everything changed.

Daddy and Dee were planning to drive down from West Virginia to visit me in Orlando, after which they'd continue to Miami to visit my sister. But Daddy hadn't been feeling well since Easter time. He had congestion in his chest and shortness of breath. He was losing weight and was extremely weak. I insisted they postpone the trip, but Daddy was determined to come anyway. Yes, he was "West by God Virginia" stubborn.

Daddy was admitted to the hospital in late May and had about a gallon of fluid drained from his right lung. Further testing confirmed that he had mesothelioma, which few in our family had ever heard of, and which all of us, initially, had great difficulty pronouncing. The doctors explained that it was a relatively rare cancer of the lining of the lung caused by exposure to asbestos, usually many years before any symptoms appear. They also said that the prognosis for this type of cancer was not good.

During the six months of his illness, I found myself wanting to call him every day and visit him as often as I could. I flew from Florida up to West Virginia at least once a month. I wanted my heart to sing again like it had so long ago on that drive and his heart was more than ready for an encore performance.

We took risks in this new Meso Lifetime that we would never have taken before. I said, "I love you" on more than one occasion. He was a reserved man, but he said it to me, too. We forged ahead with our new relationship of discovery and rediscovery. Where once our conversations had sometimes seemed forced, now I'd call him and we'd talk about everyday things—how my son, Jonathan, was doing, West Virginia football, the weather. It didn't really matter what the words were, just that we were talking.

"Daddy, how are you doing today?" I'd ask.

"Well, pretty good," he'd say. "I'm dressed and have a free day, no doctor appointments." His West Virginia drawl flowed like a gentle river through the phone lines and gave me hope. We moved from a relationship that was devoid of day-to-day details to one that addressed the most basic aspects of human life.

"Have you eaten anything today, Daddy?"

"Tried to eat some apple sauce and bacon."

"How's the pain today?"

He'd ask questions about Jonathan and me. He'd tell me he liked it when I visited. This was big, *real* big.

As I watched Dee, his wife of almost 40 years, take care of him during those difficult six months, I saw the fruits of that commitment and stability. I was amazed by his positive attitude as I watched him struggle in the morning just to find enough energy to get dressed and yet still be able to say, "It's a pretty good day today." If I were dying, would I be so positive? I was stunned by his persistence and dedication to living when, only a couple of weeks before he died, he insisted on driving to the airport to pick up my sister. Given the same circumstances, could I have been as strong?

I was discovering who my Daddy really was, and I liked what I saw. Others already knew what I had yet to learn. "Joe was a simple man," Reverend Okey Harless was later to say at the funeral. "A simple man of faith." I thought about that a lot. I knew that the preacher was referring to religious faith, something that I'd abandoned a long time ago.

Joe, my daddy, *was* a simple man. Now I suspect that only a "simple" man could keep a smile on his face despite the intense pain. Only a "simple" man could forego bitterness about the unfairness of life and graciously accept the cards he's been dealt. Only a "simple" man could maneuver through his shortened lifetime with so much courage. In his simplicity, it appeared that Daddy had somehow figured out the meaning of his life.

Pleasure for Daddy and for the rest of our family increasingly became defined by his lack of pain and by little things, like sitting around on a Sunday afternoon reminiscing about old times. Routine was important as well. He still played the lottery every week, read the sports pages in the newspaper, watched the 11 o'clock news. Daddy chose to live his shortened lifetime just as he had before ... well, not quite.

My sister was visiting him one weekend when our mom called. It wasn't planned, but my sister ended up putting Daddy on the phone with her. They had not spoken for many years. My mom told us later what a good conversation they'd had.

"Just wanted to say I'm thinking of you," my mom said. "And if there's anything I can do."

"Thanks, Carole," Daddy said. "It's been a long time."

"We were young back then," she said. "Now we have grandchildren."

"Yes, we're lucky," he said. "And I don't have any hard feelings towards you."

"Me neither," she said. "We did our best. Take care of yourself."

And, so, a much longer lifetime was condensed into a few minutes and became part of the shorter, more immediate one.

Later, I realized that a miracle had occurred: Daddy and I accomplished in six months what we hadn't been able to do in almost forty years. We re-connected and acknowledged our love for one another. My rediscovered daddy inspired me to embrace fortitude, patience, and dignity, to seek a simple life, not to run from it. In these things, he found strength, and through those months of watching Daddy live his life to the end, they have become my goals as well.

He spent the last week of his life in Hubbard Hospice House in Charleston, West Virginia, a beautiful place on top of a mountain. He was coherent enough the day before he died to ask for each of his four daughters by name. We all arrived in time to say goodbye. Actually, he waited for us, his patience still evident.

As I drove away from Hubbard Hospice House one last time on that cold, November day, I hummed *Jack O' Diamonds*. And then it occurred to me. Maybe the Jack of Diamonds isn't an unlucky card after all. Maybe it's just another card that we all draw at some point in our lives. It's how we play it that matters. Daddy played it brilliantly.

The author is Manager of Communications for the American Automobile Club's National Headquarters in Heathrow, Florida. She has published essays in the Orlando Sentinel and articles in AAA member publications. Her short story, "Blue Impala," was a finalist in Glimmer Train's "Short-Story Award for New Writers" 2004. The author has taught at the University of Central Florida and high-school English in New York. She lives in Winter Park, Florida.

All Joking and Kidding Aside
Roberta Gordon Silver

My brother Gerald's sense of humor brought fresh air into our family gatherings. He smoothed over crises and cajoled others into better moods. While everyone else expressed negative emotion without a qualm, he grinned and entertained with anecdotes that brought smiles and chuckles from the grimmest faces. Gerald was the first male to compliment my looks and raise my self-esteem. He taught me to drive. Gerald was a hero to me.

After serving four years as a flight navigator in the Air Force during the Korean War, Gerald became an air traffic controller. But he hated the constant tension and drama, so he went to college to study auditing. After graduation he married an attractive girl from St. Louis and moved with her to Texas for his first job as an auditor for a large corporation. They produced four children in rapid succession. But he was away from home too much and his wife's solo effort of caring for four active young children strained their marriage. They moved to California and because of the distance he lived from Kansas City, none of us saw Gerald and his family very often. However, each time they came home on holidays, everyone enjoyed Gerald's easy smile, joking way and soft drawl.

In 1989, I moved to northern California and saw him more often. On a visit to his home, I was shocked to learn his daily routine. Although he traveled less than before, he had a killer commute to Los Angeles from their home in Riverside, over ninety miles. His wife was still coping with everything by herself. He couldn't enjoy his swimming pool and spa because the weekends were filled with catch-up activities. He lost his job, and this ended his marriage.

In the aftermath of that disaster, Gerald seemed content. He didn't complain. I was unaware of a health problem until one day when he was unable to walk on the beach with me at Santa Cruz. He panted and leaned against a boulder. He rested until he could catch his breath, then told me of another incident related to his breathing. On a recent vacation with his new lady friend, he'd had trouble while snorkeling in the ocean. "The instructor said we had to be able to swim," he recounted, "but he also asked if either of us smoked." He grinned and lowered his voice. "We said no, and he let us dive. Guess it was a mistake because my chest tightened. I almost didn't make it to the surface. Thought I was going to die." When I suggested he see a doctor, he refused.

I didn't hear from him for many months. Through family gossip, I learned he'd sold the Riverside house and bought a home in Dallas. For the next two years, he worked less and worried more, borrowing from relatives to hang onto his house. His efforts failed and he lost it in foreclosure. Defeated, he drove to Kansas City to live with our aged and grumpy father. Gerald began drinking to excess and finally Dad booted him out.

During the next several months I saw him a couple of times. He and his latest girlfriend moved to Fresno, where the cost of living was lower and where there was a Veteran's Hospital, important because he had no medical insurance. One day I received another call from him. The ever-cheerful Gerald surprised me when he said, "I've been a little under the weather."

With prodding, I learned he'd been diagnosed with small cell carcinoma of the lungs. He explained he'd already started chemotherapy and he was on the road to recovery. I didn't know what to say. I agreed to be there the following week. As soon as our conversation ended, I telephoned various family members. My sister, Adrienne, decided to fly to California to join me. I appreciated the moral support. On the one hand, we worried about Gerald, but on the other, because of his assurances, we thought it might not be too serious.

Adrienne and I arrived at his house on a beautiful day, carrying gifts of huge artichokes and almonds we'd purchased on the road. The door flew open and my brother sprang out, laughing and dancing a jig. He clowned with facial grimaces, dressed in a robe, with a bright red woolen cap on his head.

"Wanted you to see what a sick person looks like," he joked, as if daring us to think he was ill. Closing the door after ushering us into the foyer, he pulled off the hat to reveal a bald head. It was a shock to see his shiny pate.

Adrienne and I hugged him. She said, "You're as handsome as ever."

His girlfriend took over as hostess and Gerald went to his bedroom. He returned dressed in slacks and a shirt, a small boating hat resting on his head. Gerald played the hospitable host and wined and dined us with good cheer. We reminisced about early life in the Gordon household. After the meal, we all went out to the patio and both my brother and his friend smoked with their coffee.

I was stunned. "You're still smoking!"

Gerald raised an eyebrow. In a defensive tone, he said, "My doctor didn't say I couldn't."

Then we discussed his treatment. The course of chemo was already over, he told us, and the doctor saw no more cancer on the X-rays.

"So, you see, I'm cured."

I needed to believe him.

Adrienne and I left Fresno with warm feelings. She returned to the East Coast and I got on with my life. Neither of us worried much about our brother; his optimistic attitude was contagious. I heard no more for three months, until Gerald called to tell me he was moving to Long Beach to live with his daughter, Denise. He'd also be near another VA hospital. He said the cancer had returned and had spread through his body.

A couple of weeks passed. Gerald called and asked me to come see him. He said he was bored and wanted company. I made arrangements to be off work for a week and drove south, not knowing what to expect. Denise and her husband made him feel welcome in their small apartment. She had a part time job as a nurse with flexible hours that summer, so she could look after her father.

Gerald had lost an alarming amount of weight in the three months since I'd last seen him. In the week I spent there, I saw dramatic changes in Gerald's condition. I thought it odd that no one spoke about taking things one day at a time. His daughter talked about Gerald's future plans as if he'd be up and about like his former self in no time, even though one of Gerald's other children told me his new doctor had said the cancer had spread to his bones, brain and liver. The doctor had told Gerald to get his affairs in order very soon.

I wondered about it to my nephew. "Gerald's making plans to go places next fall. Doesn't he understand he's dying?" He replied, "No. He gets mad if anyone suggests anything negative."

Denise added, "I think if he admitted he was dying, he'd curl up into a ball and wouldn't come out of it."

I went off to bed but couldn't sleep. A wave of anger washed over me. *How could Gerald be so stupid? Why didn't he check out his lungs years ago when he was short of breath?* He waited too long.

When the anger passed, I wondered if Gerald had ignored the truth to avoid dealing with it. After hours of tossing and turning, I saw it another way. Maybe it wasn't that Gerald was incapable of dealing with the truth. Maybe Gerald wanted to protect everyone else by encouraging others around him to stay positive.

With each passing day, Gerald weakened. Denise reluctantly ordered a hospital bed from a medical supply rental company. She may have thought Gerald might get angry because he'd made such an effort to avoid looking like an invalid, sitting up fully dressed at all times. Nevertheless, the bed was set up in the living room that afternoon and Gerald didn't object.

Toward the end of the week, he roused himself to speak in a serious tone to his daughter. Gazing intently at her he said, "I'm a goner, aren't I?" Stunned, she couldn't speak. Then she nodded. He held her hand and closed his eyes.

The next day Gerald was moved to the hospital, where he could be made more comfortable. An ambulance arrived to transport him. He showed calm acceptance. Quietly, he thanked the paramedics when they carried him down the stairs.

The following day, I visited him for the last time. Amidst the odors of starched linen and antiseptic, Gerald lay propped in bed carrying on conversations with each of his children. The telephone rang. Our brother Arthur, living in Houston, had just returned from an extended trip to Europe.

As my brother spoke to Arthur, he smiled. His voice was clear. Instead of complaining, he asked questions about Arthur's trip. Like a good host, when he hung up with Arthur, Gerald tried to make each of us all feel comfortable. He'd put aside all joking and kidding, but remained the cheerful Gerald he had always been to us.

Two weeks later, alone in his room in the night, his life ebbed away.

A former teacher and counselor with degrees in Special Education and Counselor Education, Roberta is a member of the Missouri Writer's Guild and is the author of numerous published articles, two essays published in anthologies by Maril Crabtree entitled *Sacred Stones and Sacred Fire* and an historical novel entitled *Voices of Eternity*.

In Search of a
Simpler Time
Nancy Harless

We were partners in crime. What started as mischief became a rit-
ual we looked forward to every Christmas. It felt deliciously
wicked, even more so because we were doing it secretly.

There were more children than money in our large family, but
every year our parents managed to make Christmas a celebration
to be remembered. Sugar cookies were baked and decorated to
resemble tiny trees and candy canes. The extended family drew
names for gift exchanges. Every year, we waited excitedly for the
mailman to bring a box stuffed full of presents from cousins from
distant places. Every year a box from a foreign land called
Minnesota arrived smelling of sweet, hickory bacon butchered,
smoked and cured by our grandfather. Yes, we had traditions that
remained unchanged year after year and could be counted on as
sure as the sun rising in the morning. They were part of the season and part of our Christmas.

But one of my fondest Yuletide memories is the secret I shared
only with my older sister, Barbara. Our crime was committed
while we were supposed to be shopping for our siblings. Before we
were old enough to earn our own money, our father would give us

each five dollars one week before Christmas. With the money came stern instructions that it was to be spent only on presents for our sisters.

Our parents would load us into our old car. We would bump and lurch down the road to the nearest town where they would drop us at the door of the dime store. The crisp bill given to me by my father was folded and put away safely in my pocket. I checked for it frequently and felt a quick rush every time I reached into my pocket as I planned all the wonderful surprises I would buy.

I took my shopping seriously. A tiny bottle of Evening in Paris perfume for Joyce. To my six-year-old tastes it smelled heavenly and looked sophisticated in its royal blue bottle. A hefty bottle of bubble bath for Barbara with a picture of a gardenia on the front. I smiled when I imagined her up to her neck in a bathtub full of bubbles. For Pammy, a colossal bottle of blowing bubbles was the perfect choice, but I would have to blow the bubbles for her, since she was just a baby.

Once our shopping was completed Barbara and I would sneak to the soda counter. We would climb up on the tall round stools, plunk down our leftover change and count to see if we had enough. We always did. Grinning from ear-to-ear, we proudly ordered hot fudge sundaes. As we sat there, conspirators in crime, skinny legs dangling, we giggled and licked the thick, gooey chocolate from our spoons. This tradition began when Barbara was nine years old and I was only six. It continued through our high school years. No one in our family ever discovered our secret.

Fast-forward fifty years. Barbara was diagnosed with lung cancer. Later the disease spread to other parts of her body. I left my Midwest home to care for her during treatment. Because it had spread to her brain stem, her doctor told us there was no cure, but palliative therapy would allow her more time to live. She chose to undergo the horrendous treatments needed to extend her life. First she endured radiation. Every day for several weeks, particles of energy bombarded her brain. Fatigue and nausea became her daily companions. Next, chemotherapy began with all its unpleasant side effects. However, after a few weeks, with the help of new medications, we were pleasantly surprised to find that Barbara no longer experienced nausea. Her appetite even returned.

That is when we began our quest. We were determined to find the perfect match for the sundae of our childhood memory. The ice cream must be the hard kind, the harder the better, since the thick, hot fudge would cause it to melt right away. And it had to have a cherry on top. And don't even think about trying to serve us in a paper container. No, it absolutely must be in a glass dish shaped like a tulip. That was the recipe. We spent the entire time she was in treatment in search of the absolutely perfect concoction. We didn't tell anyone else what we were doing; once again it was our secret.

Treatment day was always Monday; by evening she could barely keep her eyes open. The week became a blur of growing fatigue, confusion and weakness, but by the weekend, Barbara would begin to rally and by Sunday she was ready.

"You think we will find it this time?" she'd ask. We'd laugh and then climb into the car and off we would go.

We ate a lot of ice cream that year, but something was always slightly off-kilter. Soft ice cream wasn't the same as the hard-pack we remembered, chocolate syrup didn't give the same sensual thrill as the thick goo of our childhood delight, or the cherry on top was missing, or even worse, it was served in a paper container. The exact replica seemed impossible to find. Week after week we searched for the perfect combination. We were on a mission, in search of a shared childhood memory and a happier time.

Her treatments were coming to an end and soon I would need to return to my home and leave my sister, for a time, in the capable hands of other family members. But we had not accomplished our mission.

"We didn't find it this year, did we," Barbara commented with a sigh one morning. I knew exactly what she meant.

"No, but we're not giving up!" I replied, remembering reading about an old-fashioned ice cream parlor about one hour away, touted to have "the best ice cream in the world." "Are you up for a road trip?"

The following day we loaded ourselves into the car and bumped down the road. It was a long trip for Barbara, much longer than any we had previously attempted. By the time we arrived at the 1950's-decorated ice cream parlor, she was drained. She needed help just to get out of the car.

"Are you sure that you're up for this today?" I asked.

She smiled weakly and nodded her head, "This looks good. It just might be the place."

As the waitress held out menus, Barbara spoke softly. "We won't need those. We already know what we want: hot fudge sundaes. Do you use hard ice cream?"

"Of course," the waitress replied.

Barbara beamed at me. "I think that we might have found it." The waitress gave us a puzzled look then scribbled our order on her notepad.

Soon she returned carrying two tall tulip-shaped glasses filled with cold, hard vanilla ice cream smothered in rich, thick hot fudge sauce, topped with a squirt of whipped cream and a cherry. "Is this what you wanted?" she asked as she plunked them down on the counter.

I turned toward my sister. Our eyes locked. The silent, secret question hung in the air between us. Was it? We looked at the sundaes. We slowly picked up our spoons, plunged them into the sweet, cold confection and brought them to our mouths. As I licked the thick, rich chocolate goo from my lips, I looked toward Barbara and saw that she was doing the same. We smiled and then giggled. Mission accomplished.

There we were, not two overweight, middle-aged women enjoying an afternoon dessert with more calories than either needed, but two giggling little girls, perched on high stools, skinny legs dangling, sharing the precious bond of sisterhood, carried back to a time when life was simple and "palliative treatment" were words that had no meaning for us.

It's been three years since my sister died. While the progression of grief has been defined by some as having five stages, my own didn't fit neatly into any sort of sequence. It began on the day of Barb's diagnosis. I am a nurse: my knowledge base didn't allow me to linger long on either cancer of the lung or its metastasis to the brain stem: I knew what the outcome would be. I shot through those first two stages in about five minutes, and then swung wildly between bargaining and anger for months.

I bargained among the family to support my sister, financially and emotionally, so that she might remain in her home. I bargained with God to give Barbara just one more summer with her roses and gardens. Our family granted my wish. God didn't.

I moved into my sister's home to become her primary caregiver, and I became fiercely protective. Behind her back, I raged. I raged at everyone and everything—doctors, nurses, healthcare systems, social and religious institutions—but most ashamedly, I raged at my own family members who, in my clouded perception, weren't providing enough support. I raged at a God who would randomly choose whose life would be lived easily and whose would not. And I raged inwardly, full of self-loathing and helplessness, because there was absolutely nothing I could do to stop my sister's impending death.

Toward the end, when the cancer had progressed to the point where maintaining her life would simply be a farce—a body that no longer contained my fun-loving sister, I, with a medical power of attorney, permitted all treatment, save pain control, to be stopped.

Was it a difficult decision? No. Over many a night spent not sleeping, Barb had made it clear. For her, life was much more than just breathing. During one particular conversation held in the wee morning hours, I recall her asking for my help. "I don't want my boys to have to make the hard decisions. You're going to have to do it. And don't let them keep me around longer than I'd want too, you know?" Then, with the style so typical of my sister, who used humor to get through anything difficult, she threw her head back, laughed and said, "I mean, a lady knows when it's time to go."

I think about my sister at odd times. Certain things trigger vivid memories—peacock feathers, French manicures, clothes that glitter, soul music, the cinnamon scent of warm sticky buns, and hot fudge sundaes are among a few. Most of the time, when I remember, I don't feel sad. Barbara died much like she had lived, struggling, but, indeed she was a lady—a very strong, beautiful lady.

Nancy Leigh Harless is a retired nurse practitioner who enjoys volunteering, traveling, and writing about those experiences. She has been a contributor to several anthologies and professional journals. Nancy's first book, *Womenkind: Connection and Wisdom 'Round the World*, will be published in 2007.

Part V
LEARNING

Don't believe in miracles; depend on them.

—*Lawrence J. Peter*

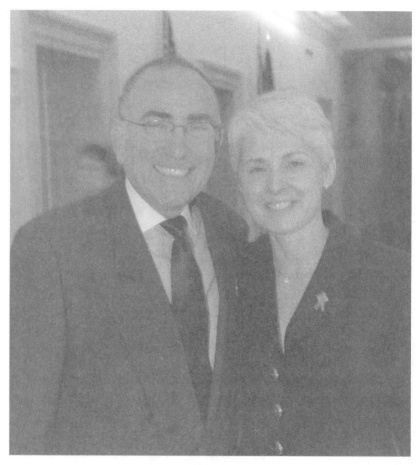

Ed and Linda Levitt, page 33

No Room for Blame

Jamie Young

When I taught school, one of the most important things that I tried to instill in my kids was empathy, caring for others and looking at the world through someone else's eyes without judgment. My three-year-old is one of the most empathetic people I know. He teaches me something new every day. He loves everyone and has a true concern for their feelings. It doesn't matter what they look like, what they do for a living, what their bad habits are or how old they are. He wants them to be happy and feel good. I sure wish we could all see the world that way.

When I was diagnosed with lung cancer, the negativity that surrounded it terrified me. Some people honestly feel lung cancer victims who smoked deserve what they get. To me, that's extremely unfair and unkind.

I can promise you that I didn't bring this on myself, and I wouldn't wish this awful disease on anyone. Smoking is a terrible addiction and a hard habit to break. Unfortunately, this is not a perfect world and we are not perfect people and of course, hindsight is 20/20. But, I can tell you this. The lung cancer patients whom I have met have been some of the most considerate and caring human beings I have ever crossed paths with. They don't deserve the physical pain and anguish of not knowing whether they will be alive tomorrow or the next day. Nobody deserves that. No matter what they have done in the past, they deserve the chance to live and be cured just as much as the next sick person.

Adults can learn a lot from children. Like them, we can be forgiving and we can be empathetic. What carefree and happy people we would be.

Jamie Young resides in Memphis, Tennessee with her husband, Jon and her son, Ryan. A graduate of the University of Mississippi, she has served as a band director at Nettleton Public Schools in Mississippi and Wooddale Middle School in Memphis. She volunteers with the Wings Foundation, hosts a fundraiser each year called "Playing for a Cure," a middle and high school band and solo competition that helps fund lung cancer research and participates in numerous lung cancer support groups including lchelp.org and lungcancersurvivors.org.

Ben and the Snow Storm

Kay Cavanaugh

The driving storm that blanketed the narrow mountain roads with snow made for a grueling journey. But my patient Ben was low on his pain medicine and the thought of him sitting in this storm with no one but his loyal old dog Bo kept me from canceling the trip.

I have been a nurse in this Blue Ridge Mountain town for 20 years. Ben, age eighty, was referred to me by his surgeon. Ben was recovering from the removal of a lobe of his right lung. He had decided against chemotherapy or radiation, letting nature take its course. "Doc told me the cancer already spread to my bones," Ben had told me. "Ain't no sense in filling this old body with poison." I had to agree.

Ben lived in an old, dilapidated house perched far up on a mountainside. As the trip wore on I questioned my decision to keep the appointment. My windshield wipers weren't working fast enough to clear the falling snow and I ended up driving with the window down, my arm stretched around to the windshield, trying to brush the icy snow from the glass as I drove. My arm turning numb, I could barely keep ahead of the snow as it distorted my view of the fast-disappearing road. I had been up that mountain 'holler' several times before, but with no road signs for miles and the heavy snowfall it was hard to recognize any familiar reference points on the way to Ben's place.

I drove until the road abruptly ended at an empty, snow-filled field. I gathered the supplies I needed to change his surgical dressing, took a deep breath and stepped out into at least four feet of packed snow. Barely able to make out anything in the distance, I trudged up the hillside towards Ben's house with the bitterly cold wind biting at my cheeks. The snow filled my boots and my toes were starting to go numb. The wind whipped up the powdery snow, obscuring my view. I tried to remember the symptoms of hypothermia; I was sure being disoriented was one of them, and I began to feel that now.

Another thirty minutes through the blizzard and I reached a house that was unrecognizable in the drifts, promising myself that if Ben didn't live there I was going to give nursing care to whoever did. I stamped my numb and stinging feet on the wooden porch and brushed off the rest of the snow from my boots with a tattered old broom that was leaning against the door.

I pounded on the door. "Ben, it's your nurse," I called. Ben responded, "Come in out of that weather, darling."

I stepped inside and Bo greeted me by slamming his large, bedraggled hindquarter against my legs, almost knocking me off my feet. The smell of burning wood from Ben's black potbellied stove filled my dripping nose. After the bitter chill outside it was hot, almost suffocating, in the little house.

Ben lived out his life in two tiny rooms. The parlor was furnished with a day bed, a rocking chair, the wood burning stove and two kerosene lamps, with two windows covered by pumpkin-colored plastic curtains. Several handmade quilts I had given him lay on the day bed. The second room, even smaller than the first, had an undersized sink and a small icebox that used ice blocks to keep his food cold. A shelf of warped plywood held his food supplies along with two cracked brown ceramic plates, two battered aluminum pots, one black metal skillet and a few assorted utensils. On the wall of the parlor facing his chair was the room's only decoration: an old picture of his parents on their wedding day, yellowed with age and set in an old brass frame. The wooden floors were old, cracked and uneven.

Soon the room felt deliciously warm and the snow in my hair and on my eyelashes started to melt. Ben looked me over and said in the voice of a father telling his young one what to do, "Take them boots off and prop them up against the stove to dry… socks too."

It was an unusual way to be greeted by a patient, but I needed to get those frozen boots off if I wanted to keep my toes. Ben took my wet socks and draped them across the stove. There was a hiss as Ben flipped them back and forth like he was frying an egg and soon the odor of cooking wool filled the room. I hoped he wouldn't order me to take off my wool slacks, even though they were soaking wet.

At first glance, Ben looked content and comfortable. A full head of thick white hair matched his full beard. His ruddy cheeks made his smile bright. His sky blue eyes twinkled when he spoke. "I didn't expect you to come out in this here storm, Kate," he said. "You know me better than that," I replied. "A little bit of snow wouldn't keep me from seeing you."

Once my hands were warm enough, I removed his dressing to reveal a bright pink, nicely healing surgical site. The incision line was a long one, starting at his breastbone and extending halfway around his back. I cleaned the site with an antiseptic, applied antibiotic ointment and covered it with a fresh, sterile dressing. With my stethoscope, I listened to his clear breathing while in my bare feet, a first in nursing care for sure, I thought to myself with a smile. I counted his antibiotics and pain medicines, and refilled the bottles from my stock supply.

"How are you feeling Ben?" I asked.

"Fine darling," replied Ben, "Bo and me, we are doing just fine."

Ben's prognosis wasn't good. The cancer had spread into his lymph nodes and bones. His time was limited and he knew it, but he was at peace with his condition. "Just gonna wait it out," he had told me before. "The old man with the sickle is gonna have to come fetch me, I ain't gonna go looking for him."

"Are the pills keeping the pain at bay?"

"Oh, now don't you go fretting about me and pain," he said. "At my age, everything is gonna give you a pain every now and then. I figure there are people a lot worse off than me. Look at the poor children starving. Their bellies pain them more than this cancer will ever pain me."

"Ben," I said, "I want you to tell me if the pain medicines stop working, OK?" I knew they would not help as his cancer spread over time. "I tell you everything Kate," he answered. "You know more about me than Bo. I just thank the good Lord for your help." I felt a tug at my heartstrings. I had grown fond of this old man and was pained that he did not have long to live.

"It's a privilege to help you, Ben," I told him. "I want you to drink more liquids and keep a pail of water close to the stove to put some moisture into the dry air. It will help you breathe easier. And if you want anything, just ask."

He took my hand, brought it to his bearded cheek. "Can you sit a spell before you gotta go back out there in that storm?"

I looked out the frosted window. It was still daylight, but the storm was not letting up. I told him, "I can stay for a while Ben, but I need to leave before the roads become invisible."

"Why shucks gal," he said jovially, "you can stay up here with me and Bo. Bo will keep you real warm." My stomach did a flip flop just thinking about Bo snuggling up to me. I was glad Ben couldn't read my thoughts. "Thanks Ben," I said, "but I need to be in town in case other patients need me."

Ben challenged me to a game of checkers, which turned into three, and he beat me each time with no effort. "Ben, you trounced me," I told him. Laughing he said, "Well I reckon I can unless the cancer gets to my brain." He glanced out the window. "Wow, look at that pure white snow piling up against the house. Like God's ice cream. Sometimes when the winds come a-howling, the snow drifts up against the doors and I can't get out."

I asked him how he spent his days and nights alone with the cold winds howling around the cracks in the doors and windows, buried in the snow.

"Most days I sit here in my rocking chair and look out the winders and watch the wild life go by. Deer roam on my little piece of land. Look out there right now, you see that doe?" I saw the beautiful animal standing close to the side of his house, looking like a picture from a greeting card. Ben joked, "I'd invite her in, but Bo doesn't like it when I look at another animal. Reckon he's jealous?" I smiled and he went on. "I never have been lonely up here. Got Bo, food to eat, things to read. What else would I want?"

Finally, I told Ben that if I wanted to make it down the mountain, it was now or never. He handed me my scorched thermal socks. They were dry and stiff. As I sat down on the edge of his bed and slipped on my socks and boots, I took another look around the rooms to see if he could use anything else to help make his days and nights more comfortable. I felt a sudden pang of pain as I realized that I would probably be the one to find him when his time came. But he had told me more than once that he wasn't afraid of death. He spoke of it as the inevitability it was that would claim us all at some point. "Ain't nothing to be scared of," he would say. "When you are dead you are dead."

Ready to go, I gave Ben a hug, Bo a pat on his shaggy head and opened the door to a whiteout. It took forty-five minutes of hard work to get back to my car. The roads were covered, icy and almost impassable. On the road, I had to stop to put chains on my tires. The ice caused my windshield wipers to freeze, and again I had to ride with the window down. The usual one-and-a-half hour drive home took four hours. I was never so happy to see my house. I dragged myself inside, peeled off the many layers of soggy clothes, and got into a hot shower. Happiness filled my tired, chilled body.

I slept well that night. As I gave in to sleep, I had a picture of Ben and Bo cuddled together in their warm house sleeping safely and comfortably and tried to figure out which of us gave the other more courage to face another day and the rest of our lives, and I smiled as I drifted off to sleep. Yes, I slept well that night in my comfortable home. And I was sure that Ben, old, in pain and facing death, was sleeping just as well in his.

A resident of Georgia, the author is a retired Registered Nurse Educator who has worked in hospitals as well as community, rural, teaching, and home health nursing. She has had 10 short stories published in various magazines.

Max's Story
Penn Wallace

"I walked away from cancer after the surgery," Max told me as we sat in the living room of his tidy White Center home. "It was like waking up from a bad dream. I look back and can't believe that it really happened to me. I've had several CT scans and X-rays since my treatment, but they were all negative. Now I don't get any regular check ups. The doctors told me that I was OK and to go away, they had sick people to deal with." These were amazing words to hear from a man who was diagnosed with terminal lung cancer in November 1994.

I have known Max for several years through our cancer support group, but I met with him on a rainy Friday afternoon to get the details of his story. When I arrived at his small home, the first thing I noticed was a stainless steel palm tree and a metal sculpture that reminded me of an Aztec temple in his front yard. In Max's post-cancer life, he has become an artist.

"I developed a terrible cough," he told me. "I generally felt bad and was coughing all the time and couldn't catch my breath. People thought I was rude, but I couldn't do anything about it. I should have known something was wrong. So I went to the clinic and they told me I had bronchitis. They took X-rays, but the tumor was behind my collar bone and they missed it."

Max suffered with this cough for about eighteen months. He was between jobs and didn't have health insurance, so he used up most of his savings covering medical bills. When he got a new job, it took several months for the insurance coverage to take effect. After the insurance kicked in, he went to a new clinic and they did another set of X-rays. "It isn't bronchitis," the doctor told him. "You have bigger problems." The doctor referred him to an oncologist for a needle aspiration, and he went there accompanied by his long-time companion, Anne.

The tests showed that Max had Stage IV lung cancer that had metastasized to his lymph system. It was around his heart, in his lungs and lining, between his lungs and in his ribs.

"It's inoperable," the oncologist told him. "I suggest that we start a regimen of chemotherapy and radiation, but the best that we can hope for is to slow down the progress of the disease."

Max asked the usual first question: "How long do I have?"

"It's hard to say, Max. Maybe six months, maybe a year."

"Do you have any guns?" the doctor asked Max. "If you have guns in the house it might be a good idea to get rid of them."

"Why?" Anne wanted to know.

"We've seen suicides after people have received this diagnosis."

Anger is the normal first stage of grief. Sometimes it is necessary to find something on which to focus that anger. Anne focused her fury on the doctor. *He doesn't know us* she thought.

"The diagnosis was a wake up call," Max remembers. "I realized that I wasn't bullet proof."

The oncologist treated him first with radiation, then chemotherapy. Max was given Etopside, also known as VP 16, and Cisplatinum, two very serious chemotherapy drugs. They nearly killed him. He was sick all the time. He barely had enough energy to go from the couch to the bathroom. When he did manage to drag himself to the bathroom, he spent hours bent over the toilet vomiting. They gave him nausea pills that cost twenty-five dollars each, but they did no good. He could not hold them down and the pills always ended up in the toilet.

To complicate the problem, Max has had diabetes for thirty years. He takes insulin several times a day. Since Max could not hold down what little he did manage to eat, it caused a real problem for his diabetes. During his cancer treatment he became the fire department's best customer, as they had to revive him several times. Anne had to force honey down him just to get some sugar in his system and she learned to give him emergency injections.

Max always had a bushy mustache, but after the chemo he had about five hairs on each side of his nose. His once-long hair fell out so he wore scarves to cover his head. When he was well enough to leave the house, he drove to a gas station to fill up and the owner told him they did not allow gang members and that they would not serve him. Max didn't have the energy to argue and just left. To this day Max won't go back there.

To everyone's surprise, the treatment worked. The tumors shrank enough that the oncologist referred Max to a thoracic surgeon. "Dr. Krutcher told me that he wouldn't waste his time on me," Max remembers. "If I didn't quit smoking, he wouldn't perform the surgery." Max had tried to quit smoking for years, but couldn't. The chemo did the trick for him. He was so sick during the therapy that he couldn't smoke. When he finished the chemo, he never touched another cigarette.

"When I was growing up," Max told me, "smoking cigarettes was cool, it was fashionable. Lung cancer isn't fashionable."

"I wanted to know what my alternatives to surgery were," Max went on. "They said there weren't any, I was going to die. I might not wake up from surgery or I might live another six months, but my life was over. But I had to at least try, I couldn't just give up."

"We wanted to get a second opinion," Anne said. "We went to this real expensive doctor that we had to pay for ourselves. The doctor had worked as a Ferrari mechanic to pay his way through medical school. He and Max got to talking about cars. I just kept looking at my watch and thinking, what is this costing us." The second doctor confirmed the diagnosis: Max's only hope was to remove the tumors surgically, but it was only postponing the inevitable.

Max scheduled the surgery and then the nurses went on strike. They could not do the operation without nurses, so the operation was postponed. Without the operation, Max would have died, but luckily the nurses settled the strike before Max's surgery date.

"It was a total fluke that I got Dr. Krutcher," Max went on. "He was one of the top thoracic surgeons in the country. Things just came together; it was like the Perfect Storm. Here I was a pauper without health insurance, then I got a new job and their insurance sent me to a world-class surgeon, the chemo and radiation worked and the surgery worked. I hadn't done any good deeds to deserve this. They took out half of my left lung, two ribs and part of my lymph system. They had to cut the artery that goes to my left lung, so it doesn't put oxygen in the blood, it's like I only have one lung. Every breath I take is a good breath."

After the surgery, the doctors gave Max morphine to ease the pain. Afraid of becoming addicted, Max would not take the drug. Anne told me that he picked up the prescriptions and threw them in the vegetable drawer in the refrigerator. When they told the doctor about this he replied, "If you survive, then we'll worry about the addiction."

"When I was diagnosed," he told me, "I thought that my life was over, but I got a second chance. Only those that have been there can possibly understand the gravity of the situation. I realized that money meant nothing. I could have won the Power Ball lottery and it wouldn't have bought me anything. In life there are so many things that rich people can buy their way out of, drunken driving tickets, murdering their ex-wife and her boyfriend, but no amount of money can buy you even one more day when you get a terminal cancer diagnosis."

By the 4th of July, Max had started improving. He and Anne were going to dinner at Max's mom's house and he felt like riding his motorcycle for the first time. He lost control and crashed crossing some railroad tracks. The chemo and radiation had made his bones so weak that Max ended up with a broken collar bone. The bone would not heal and he had to have it replaced with a stainless steel collar bone.

Anne had moved in with Max to take care of him. Max's mom and sisters came over during the day to look after him and Anne took care of him after work, as he needed twenty-four hour care. At one point, Anne had to quit her job to be there for Max.

"It's been a wild ride," Anne told me. "It's been emotional surfing; I had waves of compassion, anger, resentment. We have become a one income family. The disease ate up most of our savings." She says that she wakes up in the middle of the night worrying about losing Max and what life would be like without him. "When I first met Max, he was like a side of beef, bulging biceps, abs. It's been hard to see his body change so drastically. I look at his body, how he was cut open, and the staples that they used to close him up. It was amazing. Everything about a person changes, physically, emotionally, mentally, the caregiver sees that. That's not the person you hooked up with."

At first the doctors gave Max six months, then one year, then two years, then he kept on living. He put everything in order and got ready to die, then they had to shift gears.

"He shouldn't be here," Anne says, "but he's going to live. I know it sounds bad, but I kept thinking *when are you going to die?*"

Anne thumbed through the notebook that they kept during Max's treatment. It is a record of all the things they went through. "Max has changed since the diagnosis," she told me. "He is really smart, he has a lot of interests in mechanics, art and how things work. He doesn't care what people think about him, he's kind of offbeat. I am really surprised that he goes to the Cancer Support Group. Sometimes he can't handle the emotions. Getting too close to the people in Group is a constant fear for Max. When we lose a member, it takes a huge emotional toll on him. Sometimes he can't go because he is too distraught."

Anne told me of living with cancer, "You find out who you really are. Max was never the kind of person who would have had cats. But after the cancer, a big black and white cat started hanging around the house and they bonded. Shortly after, we adopted a Russian Blue and now Max is a cat man. We have become introverted since the illness," Anne said. "We don't feel the need to go out and socialize."

"I can't be around smoke anymore," Max says. "Anne still smokes, I make her go outside to smoke, but when she comes in I can't stand to be around her. There is so much that changes. Anne had dealt with alcohol before, but since my illness she has stopped drinking."

Since the cancer, Max still deals with depression. He can no longer surf; he doesn't have the lung capacity. When he gets depressed, he goes out and works in his shop. He worked part time for five years after the surgery, to help out his employer. Then he got pneumonia and had to quit and go on full disability. "I had to stop worrying about my boss and start worrying about myself," he said.

"I have to play it as it comes. I can't change it. Now I take life gently. I still have three bikes. I miss my income but my time is my own. When I was trying to work one day a week I had to be in bed by nine every night and the next day I was dead. I was tired for five years. Now I'm going to spend whatever time I have left doing what I want to do."

Max sat back and surveyed his living room, smiling past Anne to the rainy afternoon outside.

"There is so much to enjoy, you'll find it if you give yourself a chance."

Penn Wallace is a graduate of the University of Oregon. He received his MBA in management information systems at City University in Seattle, WA. His writing has appeared in *Nor'Westing Magazine* and *Good Old Boat* and elsewhere. He and his wife, a cancer survivor, are members of the Group Health Cancer Support Group in Seattle. He currently lives in the Seattle area with his wife and two daughters.

Continued from page (140)

Where to Seek Treatment

If your case is unusual, if there is some doubt about the best possible option for you to pursue, or if you require technology or a special drug that is not available in your geographical area, then a large, major metropolitan medical center may be right for you, despite its distance from your home. However, if the treatment can be done locally, that is probably your best option. You can always go back to the major medical center periodically for follow-up by their physicians, especially if you are in an experimental study or special treatment protocol. The local oncologist, if he is the type of physician that I described above, will have no reservations about working with the specialist at the medical center to get your therapy accomplished. You should also know that many major medical centers have recognized the undesirable medical effects of making ill patients travel long distances and have opened up satellite units in smaller suburban and rural areas.

Continued on page (188)

How My Mother's Lung Cancer Has Affected Me

Emily Monroe

How has my mother having lung cancer affected me? The question has been put to me many times, and I've come up with many different answers. The complete answer though, is a simple one: lung cancer affects everything. My mom's lung cancer has and continues to affect and impact my life completely.

When I was thirteen years old, my mom was diagnosed with Stage IV lung cancer and my life was turned upside down. I was young, confused and scared. After a time of nerve-racking tests and stressful waiting, she was told to go home and spend the remaining six to eight months of her life with her daughters.

Well, if you knew my mom you would know that this news didn't settle well with her. As a stubborn risk-taker and independent woman, she looked for a second opinion. God led her to Vanderbilt Medical Center in Nashville, Tennessee. My mom is now a very active patient advocate at Vanderbilt and she has been the subject of numerous newspaper articles and TV interviews, including *The Wall Street Journal* and a *LiveStrong* survivor video. There are many stories of how my brave and courageous mother fought and defeated her cancer and then fought again. To sum it up, over five years, consisting of five surgeries and a year of chemotherapy, with the help of some loving and caring doctors, nurses, friends, family, and of course the miracle of prayer, God healed my mother and today she is cancer free!

Some people are surprised by just how much something like this can take over and change your whole life. Above all, I learned that with the help of God anything is possible. My mom is living proof that no mountain is too high and no road is too rough for us. She is my inspiration to get the absolute most I can get out of life because you don't know the future and you can't control it even if you did. I have learned to do everything I can to live life to the fullest.

This bump in the road has also taught me to take care of myself. So many things in today's society are unhealthy and unclean. Why take chances? I say, do as much as you can to prevent the possibility of disease.

Finally, I have learned to appreciate what I have been blessed with. My mom has been given the chance to meet and talk to many people struggling and dealing with the very same battle she fought and is still fighting today. Unfortunately, not every family's story is the same as ours. Our journey hasn't been a walk in the park; we've had our share of pain and heartache. But the only thing that matters now is that I have my mom. And I know I will never take that for granted.

Mom is a survivor and I am so proud of her. It wasn't fun, but the trial brought me closer to her. Above all, I've learned there is a reason for everything. Sometimes the hardest journeys are the most worthwhile.

Emily is the 18 year old daughter of Lori Monroe, diagnosed with Stage IV lung cancer, whose story also appears in this book. She was only 13 years old when her mother received a prognosis of 6–8 months. Since then, Emily has graduated high school with honors and now attends Western Kentucky University. She has started a not-for-profit organization called "Lori's Hope," the mission of which is to help other teens and young adults whose lives have been affected by cancer.

Continued from page (184)

What if Chemotherapy Doesn't Work?

Unfortunately, many lung cancer patients cannot have surgery, and chemotherapy or radiation therapy rarely produces a cure. When the chemotherapy or other treatment is no longer able to keep the disease from progressing, the patient and his or her family or advocate must talk about options with the oncologist and/or the patient's internist or family practice specialist. There are many things that can be done to help a patient in these circumstances.

If a patient's medical condition still allows it, the oncologist sometimes recommends trying another type of chemotherapy. Normally, after two or three different types of chemotherapy treatments, most patients are unable to endure another round with yet another drug. For that reason, while experimental drugs may also be considered, this option should only be considered if the patient is still strong enough to tolerate it. At this point, you may wish to seek a second opinion to explore options that your oncologist is not using or is unfamiliar with.

Continued on page (212)

When I Was a Little Girl

Diane Cole

When I was a little girl, there was a ride called The Roundup at an amusement park in Chicago, my home town. The riders would stand around the perimeter of a large circular enclosure and as the ride picked up speed, the centrifugal force kept you flat against the sides as the floor fell away. I never went on The Roundup, but my life after my lung cancer diagnosis was how I imagine that ride felt.

My story started with my younger sister's heart attack. She was told that her condition, which required an emergency angioplasty, was genetic. Learning this and having always been proactive about my health, I called my internist for an appointment. While she felt that, given my current health and lifestyle, heart disease would probably not be a serious issue for me, she scheduled me for a coronary CT scan.

I underwent the test the following week. As I lay on the table trying to stay calm, I thought about my stepsister, who had died from breast cancer six weeks before. She had been strong and upbeat throughout her illness and I imagined she was there with me, helping me stay calm. The next day my doctor called me with the test results. The good news was that my heart was in great shape. I thought, okay, that scare is over. Then I heard her say "But we found a spot on your left lung." From what seemed like a great distance, I heard her telling me not to overreact, that it could be an infection or tuberculosis. But I knew instinctively what it was. Somewhere deep inside myself I always knew I would have to deal with cancer at some point in my life, but I never imagined it would be so soon and I never thought it would be lung cancer. I had quit smoking twenty-five years ago.

What followed was a whirlwind of doctor appointments, another CT scan, this time of the lungs, and a PET scan. I was diagnosed with a 1.5 centimeter adenocarcinoma. I thought of Dana Reeve, another non-smoker, who had been diagnosed with lung cancer a few weeks earlier. I was in a complete state of shock.

My doctors decided that my best option was surgery, to remove the lower lobe of my left lung. At the same time, I would undergo a biopsy of the lymph nodes around the windpipe. If, after surgery, my cancer was found to be Stage I-A, without involvement of the lymph nodes, I wouldn't need chemotherapy. If cancer was found there, I would have to go through the treatment. Even with half of my left lung gone, I would retain 80% of total lung capacity. Once I recovered and got back in shape, I wouldn't notice the difference most of the time; I could live a normal life. Since my cancer was located in a so-called good spot, my surgeon was optimistic that everything would go well.

The day of surgery, the Chicago White Sox were in the World Series and the city was going crazy. As I was wheeled down a long hallway into surgery, I passed by photographs of all the previous presidents of the hospital hanging on the walls. They were all wearing Sox caps! At least I got a laugh in before the operation.

Post-op my cancer was found to be Stage II-A. One lymph node was involved, so chemotherapy was in the cards for me. And a cure was now off the table. Now I was told I had a 60%–70% chance of living past five years. I was getting scared, but I had to think positively. The good news, it was caught early and I know

now that many people with this disease are given survival rates much lower than mine.

I have to admit I never thought I would be a "graceful" cancer patient, like Dana Reeve. I never stopped thinking about her and how she was doing. She was brave, beautiful and strong. Me, I thought I was falling apart emotionally. Who were all these survivors I was reading about or seeing on morning TV shows? Where did they find the strength and fortitude? I struggled with this constantly. I went to a healer, spoke at length with a therapist in Los Angeles who had been my step-sister's lifeline and had had regular sessions with my own therapist. I felt like I had no center. I was taking Xanax every six hours but my anxiety would not go away. My friends and family were there for me, but they didn't recognize me. I didn't recognize myself. I lost weight. I needed to have the TV on to fall asleep. I'm single, but for the first time, I really felt alone. I missed my parents. I kept asking myself, what am I fighting for? I have no husband or children, what is the point? But I came to realize that being alone had its advantages: I could concentrate on myself and find what I needed to get though the next several months.

My chemotherapy was going to be four rounds, two sessions each, for a total of eight sessions. My oncologist was upbeat and positive. She told me I would do really well, since I had bounced back from the surgery so quickly and was already back on my feet. The treatment schedule would be two weeks on chemo and one week off. I was told that working during treatment might not be possible because I might feel too sick to stand on my feet eight hours a day. I'm in the retail industry, working for an international luxury goods company. I love my job and had been with the company for over 14 years when this happened. I weighed my options and decided to take a leave of absence. My company took amazing care of me. It was overwhelming when the hospital bills started coming in. Thankfully, I didn't have to worry, which I knew could be a major problem for some people dealing with serious health issues. I was lucky: I could focus on my treatment and on beating my cancer.

After my first session, I felt a huge sense of relief. I was finally fighting back. My anxiety evaporated and I stopped taking Xanax. The first two rounds went well but the last two were terrible. I became dehydrated and at one point I needed a transfusion of magnesium, which was eaten up in my body by the chemotherapy drugs. By the end of the second month, my hair started to fall out. I knew it was going to thin, but I had no idea how much I would lose. I ended up losing more than half. I had to keep telling myself it could be worse, it could be worse. I lost over twelve pounds and I avoided looking at myself in a mirror. I became depressed and felt like I was at the bottom of a black hole: I was exhausted emotionally and physically. I cried a lot. The healer I had seen had given me a sketchbook and colored pencils. She told me to start a "joy" book. I drew pictures of myself feeling great and of my favorite scenery in Costa Rica. I would look at those pictures and tell myself I just had to get through the winter. I was hibernating until spring, when all this would be behind me.

I live two blocks from the hospital. Even if I was feeling tired I made myself walk to treatment. The exception was the very last session when I was just too exhausted and sick, so I took a cab. Two of my mother's life-long friends went to every round of chemo with me. Many other people offered their support, but I felt the most comfortable with them. I have come to treasure them both and feel that they are a gift brought to me by the cancer.

I was blessed many times over with cards, phone calls and gifts from friends, family and clients. So many wanted to help with anything I might need. I tried to answer as many calls as I could, but I was just too overwhelmed. I chose to spend this time alone with a few exceptions. People who cared about me were frustrated by this. I understood, and told everyone I would call if it was necessary. Reading was difficult, the drugs made it hard to concentrate. I became obsessed with old black and white movies, and would find myself disappearing into the past, mesmerized by the costumes, sets, and dialogue. Strangely, I got very attached to the contestants on *American Idol*!

Now, at six months after treatment, I look inside myself and I am just beginning to understand how I got out of that black hole. I found strength I didn't know I had. When I was feeling 100%, I realized that I would do whatever it took if my cancer came back. There are days I completely forget I had lung cancer. I certainly don't look like I did. I've learned some tricks with my hair so I don't feel self-conscious and I'm back to being obsessive (in a good way!) about my appearance. My weight is normal and I work out two to three days a week but I've noticed I have to take it easier now. Work is going great and I have a new love for my job. Dating is my final frontier. I've gone on a couple of casual dates, but most of the time I socialize with my close friends. I've picked up my life where I left off, going to movies, dinners, traveling and parties. I don't want cancer to define me, but it's part of me now, and I'm not ashamed of it.

If my cancer should reoccur, which is always a possibility, I would do things differently. I would let more people in and lean on them more. And I found that the cliché I heard about the cancer experience was true: I don't take as much for granted anymore. Living from CT scan to CT scan, I'm learning to live life more in the moment, without sweating the small stuff. I have made some long range plans and even though I feel some trepidation about this, I need to live my life as normally as possible. It's my "new" normal. I'm realizing over and over how truly lucky I was, catching my lung cancer early. Early detection makes the difference between having a chance to survive or not. Research into treatment for this form of cancer is under-funded and the disease is under-diagnosed because of its link to smoking. Most of the public believes lung cancer to be self-inflicted because of smoking. I want to help change that. When I pass a young girl smoking on the street, I want to stop and tell her my story.

Cancer didn't change who I am, but it brought out parts of me I didn't know existed. I wanted to be the "graceful" survivor, and I think I am. I've kept my sense of humor and I crack a not-so-politically-correct cancer joke now and then. I haven't decided where I can offer help in the fight against lung cancer but I think helping to raise awareness would be a great place to start.

A native of Chicago, Diane has worked in the fashion industry on 7th Avenue in New York City and in Chicago for over 16 years, most recently with the iconic House of Chanel. Diane lost her mother to lung cancer. Today Diane is cancer free.

David's Story

Lynn Costigan

⁓

On November 9, 2004 my husband went to the hospital for a CT scan. He had been experiencing headaches, extreme fatigue and dizziness while he was driving his truck at work. When we went back to get the results the doctor said, "You have a brain tumor." He basically told David he had about a year to live. I nearly fell to the floor as I grabbed David's hand. I remember saying, "Oh my God this can't be true." I burst into tears.

My husband screamed at the top of his lungs, "Well that's just not good enough for me. I have a wife and four children, and I am only forty-nine years old!" We walked out of the doctor's office. We drove home in tears, terrified, asking why, why, why?

My mind was filled with questions. *What did they mean he has a brain tumor?* I was paralyzed. *How can something like this happen to a loving, devoted, caring husband and father?* Frantically, I called my mom, who lives sixty miles away. She has always been there for me through the hardest of times, and I have drawn my strength from her my whole life. She was at my side in less than an hour.

David was rushed to the University of Massachusetts Memorial Hospital in Worcester. I left with my mother to pick up my sixteen-month-old son from daycare. Next, I had to explain to my twelve-year-old son Ryan that Daddy had to go to another hospital because they found a tumor in his brain. I told him that Daddy needed to see a team of special doctors who were going to help him. I called my twenty-five-year-old stepdaughter Jessica and twenty-one-year-old stepson Joshua. I told them the news about their Dad. They joined me and we raced to the hospital. I tried to remain calm and strong for them, but deep inside I was screaming with pain and fear.

Two days later, David underwent brain surgery. We waited eight hours. The surgeon finally informed us that the brain cancer had come from his lung, and that David had Stage IV lung cancer. There were twelve of us who had endured this waiting game together, and as the news spread, the room was filled with screams, tears and anger. I went to see David, but kept my visit brief so he could rest from his invasive surgery. My brother-in-law, John, drove me home. I remember his words as if they were said yesterday: "Don't worry, we will get through this. David is a fighter, not a quitter. We're going to take it one step at a time. Whatever you need, we are all here for you." When I went to bed that evening, I wrote down all my fears and asked God for his guidance and strength. I knew this was more than I could handle alone.

By Thanksgiving, my husband underwent whole brain radiation and started eight months of chemotherapy. In January, he had thirty days of radiation to the chest. In August 2005, David was told the lung tumor was no longer responding to the chemotherapy. In September he had the lung tumor removed. Following that, David was declared NED (No Evidence of Disease)!

For the last seven months David has been in remission. We are fortunate to have four beautiful children who inspired him to fight and an incredible network of family and friends who prayed constantly for him. We found a wonderful church where we met many wonderful people. David's determination and courage were a great part of his recovery. One of his favorite sayings is "I don't have time to be sick."

The greatest gift you can give someone with cancer or to his care giver is encouragement, hope and optimism. It's been seventeen months since David was first diagnosed. He has been working full time for four months and feels wonderful. I have so much admiration for my husband, who refused to quit. He never said, "I can't do it." He never complained. He valued my opinion and allowed me to be with him every step of the way.

Cancer has changed our lives. We love life now more than ever before. We make the most of each day. We cherish our children and grandchildren. We always say, "I love you."

When I look back at where we were in November 2004, I am amazed at how far we have come. We learned how to put our trust in God and pray constantly. We thank God for every day we have together. I hope David will be in a medical book of wonders someday, as he continues to defy the odds. Many people are skeptical about his prognosis and compare his story to people they have known with a similar diagnosis. Hopefully they are wrong. This is David's story, written with love, and only God above knows the final chapter.

A resident of Massachusetts, the writer was inspired to enter the medical profession by witnessing the birth of her stepdaughter's child and recently received a certificate from Phlebotomy & EKG Technician school.

Lessons from Joe

Angus Woodward

Joe was the first veteran of the Battle of the Bulge I'd ever met. Joe hardly ever talked to his wife or mine about the war, but he talked about it with me, starting one long afternoon eight years before he died of lung cancer. Never one to talk much, he didn't launch into lengthy yarns of heroic battles and front-line tragedies. I pieced together the fragments enough to figure out that after fighting through the war he'd wound up in occupied Austria, driving his lieutenant around on various errands. He found time to go hunting and brought the meat to some Austrian women he and his buddies knew. There was obviously much more to tell, but like I said, Joe was never one to talk much.

Ours was an unlikely friendship. If not for Joe, I never would have tasted fried venison or squirrel stew. I never would have thought about poor country folk surviving on stewed robins and other songbirds during the depression. I would not have known that you could wade in the river and feel around in hollow logs, then grab catfish by the mouth and haul them to the bank. I have never seen anyone else crumble cornbread into a glass of milk and eat it with a spoon. He taught me how to use a carpenter's square. Most important of all, Joe taught me a couple of important lessons about dying.

Joe was thirty-nine years my senior, a Louisiana country boy who hunted with dogs and grew vegetables on the old place where he'd grown up. When we met, I was a graduate student from up north, my neck as pale as Joe's was red. I was too young to have been to Vietnam, too old for the Persian Gulf. He worked as a lab technician at a chemical plant.

I first laid eyes on Joe when I drove to his house to pick up his daughter, Jalan, whom I later married, to take her out on a date. I remember pulling up in the driveway, where Joe was kneeling beside his pickup truck, having just removed the front bumper. We shook hands, and I first heard his heavy country accent. He took me into the garage where deer skulls, tools, and bamboo fishing poles hung on the wall. I had the same curiosity as a tourist visiting abroad, and had to listen carefully to understand what Joe was saying. I think he liked me because I asked questions about his stuff.

In 1996, Joe caught a cold from our daughter Geneva, who was just a year old. The cold turned into a cough, and the cough wouldn't go away. A visit to the doctor led to an X-ray, which showed a spot on Joe's lung. Tests turned up cancer. Joe was seventy-one by then, six years into his retirement after forty-six years at the plant. He no longer smoked, but had started at age twelve and smoked heavily well into his forties. But he was tough. Part of his stomach had been removed as a result of ulcers years earlier. One day, when he was fifty-eight, he drank some coffee, went out into the woods to chop firewood, started feeling bad, drank more coffee, chopped more wood, then went to the doctor. The doctor told him he'd had a heart attack and he needed double bypass surgery.

When the cancer was found, he was still solidly built and strong. He would hobble out in the morning complaining he was "all stove up," then go out to hunt or plant potatoes or cut grass all day.

Jalan, Geneva and I were living in New Orleans by then, but we came to Baton Rouge when Joe had surgery to remove half of one lung. Before he woke from the surgery, the surgeon told Jalan and her mother that he had gotten all of the cancer and there were no signs of metastasis. But a few months later, a lump on Joe's neck turned out to be cancerous and the radiation and chemotherapy began. The cancer continued to spread into his bones and else-where. One day Joe got out of bed and his pelvis broke, the bone weakened by a tumor. By the end of the fall of 1997, Joe was too weak and sick to do much of anything.

He could still ride out to the old place, though. One warm November day, Joe and I sat on the screened porch of a fragile old house on one side of the land on which he had grown up. Before us, the autumn sun shone down on the fields where he and his parents had grown sugarcane to turn into syrup. It blazed on the bigger house where he had spent the first 17 years of his life and on the thick piney woods where he had hunted and cut firewood.

The fields, the porch and the house behind us were just quiet and still enough for Joe to say something about the war, just an off-hand comment, maybe about how cold it had been over there in the winter of 1944. After a pause, I said something about how tough it must have been to be so far from home at such a young age. Joe told me he had been part of a mortar squad, dropping shells into a tube and watching them explode a few hundred yards away. "Sometimes you could see the bodies fly up," he murmured, shaking his head. I didn't know what to say to that. Joe just leaned forward, resting his muscled forearms on his knees. He brushed back his pale gray and red hair. "A lot of bad stuff happened over there," he said. "I guess that's why I've got *this*."

I never know what to say, and in this case it took me a few moments to see what he meant. Why didn't I jump right up and tell him that his cancer was not a punishment for what he had done in the war? I sensed that one word from me might unleash a torrent of war memories, the worst ones, the ones he hadn't told to a soul. Alone on the porch out in the country, he could have told me everything, and he wanted to. But I just sat there, unable to think of a thing to say. I checked my watch, then changed the subject.

The idea of disease as punishment goes back to the Old Testament plagues and still appears in this era of AIDS. In our age of science, we know that diseases only "punish" ill-advised human behavior: long-term alcoholism leads to cirrhosis, high-fat diets can cause heart attacks, and smoking can cause lung cancer. Rarely do we attribute a disease to pure happenstance. I and everyone else in Joe's family assumed he blamed his cancer on the cigarettes he had smoked for thirty-odd years. But he took a more biblical route and blamed some act or acts he committed in the war. And I deflected his attempt to tell me what had happened, missing a chance to put his mind at ease.

In the succeeding months I pulled back from Joe. It hurts to admit it. I avoided those still moments alone with him in which he might tell me about the war. I was afraid to hear what he might tell me, and didn't know what I would say. My one attempt at helping him to cope with his guilt was buying him a hard cover edition of *Slaughterhouse Five*, thinking Vonnegut's irreverent attitude might make Joe realize that he did whatever he did in the war only because he was caught up in history's machinations.

Sometimes loved ones die and the survivors regret not telling them certain things. In this case, I regret not letting Joe say those things he wanted to say before he died. I learned that you have to listen to and share with those you love when they are alive. Like most lessons about death, it had to be learned the hard way.

I also learned a second lesson from Joe's illness.

By March Joe was bedridden. Jackie tended to him at home, sleeping beside him at night, preparing and bringing him whatever food his intermittent appetite allowed him to eat, arranging his pillows, escorting friends and family in and out at sensible intervals, bathing him, and helping him preserve his dignity. It was admirable, selfless, exhausting work. He seemed to be near death—hardly moving, eating, or breathing—for weeks.

One morning in May, Jalan, Geneva and I said good-bye to Joe and drove back to New Orleans, planning to return in a few days. As soon as we got home, we called back and learned that he had died.

For someone like me, it was hard to know what to say to Jackie on the day the man she had married at sixteen died. I don't remember what I did say, but I think I only made a stab at saying what was on my mind. I realized that thanks to her, Joe had died a good death. I had never thought about the possibility of dying a good death. Like a lot of people, I had only thought of death as a frightening, sad, painful event. But Joe had lain there in that big comfy bed in a dimly lit, familiar room surrounded by people he loved, a calm look on his face. I suddenly knew how I hoped to die and how I hoped my loved ones would die. This second lesson in death was not as painful as the first, but like many such lessons, it came unexpectedly.

We buried Joe in the shade of a huge live oak at a little cemetery out in Livingston Parish, close to the land he knew all of his life. The skies were gray and threatening all day. But just as we drove away down a country road, the sky cracked open at the horizon, and the setting sun blazed through, coloring the undersides of the clouds. I think we all took that as a positive sign of some sort, perhaps that Joe was in a better place or somehow still with us. For me, it meant that he forgave me for holding my tongue and that I should cherish both of the lessons his death had taught me: the one about letting the dying speak their minds, and the one about dying a good death.

Angus Woodward lives with his wife and two daughters in Baton Rouge. His fiction, nonfiction and poetry have appeared in a variety of journals, including *Xavier Review, Talking River Review, Louisiana Literature, Rhino, Iowa Review, Prairie Schooner,* and many others. He teaches at Our Lady of the Lake College in Baton Rouge.

Part VI

PASSINGS

I wanted a perfect ending. Now I've learned, the hard way, that some poems don't rhyme, and some stories don't have a clear beginning, middle, and end. Life is about not knowing, having to change, taking the moment and making the best of it, without knowing what's going to happen next. Delicious ambiguity.

—*Gilda Radner*

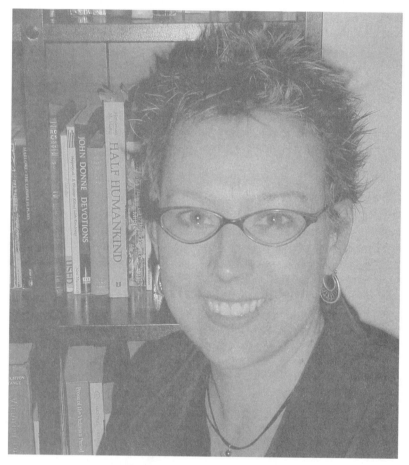

Felicia Monticelli, page 231

My Father's Last Christmas
Lorrie Kohlman

It was a snowy afternoon in mid December. On the outside, every-thing looked perfect. The powdery white landscape offered all the promise of a soft and magical holiday season. Sitting in the back seat of our family car, I usually felt so snugly warm, especially when bundled up on a crisp winter day. Today it felt different as I sat still and stared at the back of my parents' heads. Today their usual positions in the front seat had changed.

When we arrived at the mall and pulled into a parking stall, Mom shifted the car into park. She was awkward behind the wheel. Though now a weaker version of the man he had been, Dad's strength was still very much there, but from the passenger seat. There was an unspoken understanding among us that this would be our last time together in the family car. Dad's cancer continued to spread through its final stage.

Mom gave Dad a quick glance and assured him she'd be back shortly. I'm not sure how long the two of us sat there in silence, how long we both gazed out the window. When I finally looked over to Dad, he seemed so far away. I wondered where he was. What did someone in his condition think about just days before Christmas?

In the background I could hear the words to *Have Yourself a Merry Little Christmas*. The line, "Through the years we all will be together, if the fates allow" sounded so bittersweet to me that day. With each word my impatience grew, as did my realization that the holiday season would never be the same again. Any remainders of my sense of the security of childhood were slipping away with Dad.

When our eyes met in the mirror Dad looked away, but I saw his pain. I looked out the window and my eyes settled on a man holding a shopping bag. Suddenly, it hit me. Before I had time to think about what I was going to do I opened the door and jumped out, telling Dad I would be right back.

I ran towards the shopping mall. When I opened the door to the main entrance, a lifetime of memories flashed before my eyes— memories of the years gone past, of a childhood that had been spent shopping right here, within these walls.

My fondest memories were of Mom, Dad and us three kids grocery shopping here every Friday night. The highlight was when I looked up at Mom or Dad and I would ask, "Can I really have any one I want?" They would always smile and say okay. Then we three would run down the aisle laughing as we each picked out our very own box of cereal for the week. That was a big deal, and I always asked the question, because each time Mom or Dad said okay was just as exciting as the first.

After the supermarket, we'd make our way down the hall to the deli. All three of us would put out our hands for our allowance then run over to the glass jars filled with all sorts of Zout Drops. We'd eagerly scoop up piles of licorice squares, double Zout and our favorite, the Cats.

Often stopping for hamburgers on our way home, we were all ready to settle down for our family night of watching our regular Friday night TV lineup, beginning with The Dukes of Hazzard.

We all enjoyed munching on snacks and laughing at Boss Hogg's latest try at outsmarting the Duke Brothers.

Boss Hogg's laughter echoed in my memory like a fading ghost as I walked down the halls past so many stores we'd spent time shopping in. From the pet store to the bakery, the drug store to the sports store. That was where Dad took me on a few occasions to pick up the latest soccer ball. He was very proud of my drive and passion for soccer—I was his little scrapper back then.

As I took my next step, I realized the magnitude of what I was about to do. How was I ever going to find the right gift for my father to give Mom? This would be the last one ever. What was I doing? I stood in the center of the mall and took a deep breath. Again I asked myself, what would he pick? I looked in each direction until my eyes settled on the counter in the jewelry store. There, passersby were greeted with the best pieces of jewelry. I noticed a couple looking very happy as they compared rings. They were clearly starting their life together. For a moment, I felt envious that the young man still had a lifetime to become a husband and a father.

Where was I going to begin? Walking away from the happy couple towards a quiet corner, I looked down into the first sparkling showcase. There they were, staring me right in the face. I smiled as I realized just how "perfectly Dad" the gift was. I took no notice of the price, as I knew he would do the same. You can't set a value on something like this, I thought, as I stared down at the pretty lines of yellow gold forming into the shape of delicate little tulips, accented by perfectly set sapphires: Mother's birthstone.

I felt my dad's hand on mine as I paid for the gift. For the first time, I realized that I was a part of him. Never had I felt as clear about this as I did while trekking back to him. I had a new and deeper understanding of just how loved my Mother, my brother, sister and I were by him. I was really going to miss him when he was gone. But I wasn't ready to deal with that quite yet. One step at a time, and for today, I could hold onto the fact that even when the time came to let go, it wouldn't be of everything. I have always known in my heart that even though a loved one dies, the love lives on forever.

When I returned to the car with the tiny box in my pocket, I met Dad's eyes in the mirror again. This time he had that cheeky little smile in the corner of his mouth that I always hoped to see, the one he used to tease Mom with and wait for a reaction.

A few days passed and it was finally Christmas morning. I couldn't wait to show Dad what was in the mysterious box. Though I often noticed his eyes stop at the box under the tree, he never did go up to it or ask me what was in it.

I remember feeling Dad's eyes watching me as I sat curled up close to the tree. He sat back quietly on the couch while everyone passed out presents. In the midst of it all, I reached over to the little box. I met Dad's eyes, and I blinked back a tear. I needed him to know how much I loved him. I swallowed hard, and his eyes smiled at me. It was then time to turn to Mom.

She took the tiny box and noticed the looks between Dad and me. Now their eyes met, and she took a deep breath. Everyone in the room stopped and looked over. We all knew it was the last present from Dad that Mom would ever hold in her hands. Everyone waited anxiously to see what was in the box. I looked over to Dad. That glance we shared was one I will carry inside me for the rest of my life. Whatever happened after this holiday season was okay. Dad now knew how much I loved and thought of him, and that's all I needed. That was my last present to him. I knew I would hold onto this moment forever.

Mom was so touched by his gift. Dad was proud of my choice. Just then I realized the gift didn't only symbolize how I believe he loved my Mom but also how I saw him. He now knew what I thought of him. There was so much revealed inside this little box.

Each time I see those little tulips on her ears I am reminded of the day I truly became my Father's daughter. Each time I thank God for that one moment.

_____

Lorrie has spent the past fifteen years working as a staff and freelance magazine writer and editor. A resident of Canada, she is Founder and Creative Director of Kismet Kids Charitable Foundation.

Continued from page (188)

Palliative Care

For my patients who have been treated without success, I use the following benchmark to determine if he or she should go forward with a different course of chemotherapy: if the patient is able to spend half a day out of the house walking and being with the family, then that patient has enough physical strength and reserve to continue to be treated. On the other hand, because each successive new treatment for lung cancer produces less effective results and with each new treatment the wear and tear on the patient becomes more severe, I find that those patients who are so ill that they are virtually homebound or can only get out of their house in a wheelchair are not suitable candidates for additional aggressive therapy.

For patients whose lung cancer can no longer be treated, there is one type of therapy still available—palliative care. Palliative care is the science of symptom control. The patient and family or patient advocate need to consult with the treating physician about living with the illness and controlling its symptoms. Once the medical team must give up trying to shrink or eliminate the tumor, i.e., "curative" therapy, it can begin to aggressively treat the patient with a variety of drugs and technologies to minimize the discomfort of the symptoms. With the highly effective treatment options currently available to the palliative care specialist, who may be your oncologist or even your own private physician, a person can spend an extended period of time at the end of the illness, which could last many months or perhaps a year or two, in complete comfort.

Continued on page (230)

Day 1—Stage I
Tracey E. Peterkin

It's so peculiar how a tragic or life-altering event has the ability to make you keenly aware of how your life is different from those around you. Others go about their daily activities, relatively unaware that their life is passing, some happy, some miserable, most unconcerned, while *you* feel the significance of every fleeting moment. You are both disoriented and disconnected. You understand the meaning of infinite helplessness. You remember not only every meaningless detail, but it seems that all other life stops, your focus is so intense.

Neil, I remember the day in July when your cancer came back. You became ill at work and were being taken to Long Island Jewish Hospital for what we thought were kidney stones. You called: nothing serious, you said, I shouldn't worry, you loved me. I could hear your pain. I remember thinking; this was just another strange but repairable "Neil illness", one in a long line of strange but always repairable illnesses. We often joked that you were "repairable."

I lingered too long at work, which was my custom, taking a few more calls. I thought we had all the time in the world. I ignorantly believed that I needed to be at work more than you needed me. I know now that I was trying to avoid or at least shorten the inevitable hospital wait. I assured myself I would meet up with you as soon as the preliminaries were done.

You'd had pneumonia a month before and collapsed on the bathroom floor. Too stubborn and proud to call the ambulance, you made me rush home. Panicked, afraid you would stop breathing before I could get you to the hospital; I wanted to kill you; now I wonder how I could ever have had such a thought. I couldn't lift you. I just wasn't strong enough. Your breathing was shallow; your eyes were glazed from fever. My will power, terror and anger somehow combined forces and enabled me to get you to Northern Westchester Hospital.

Now, only four weeks later, you were down again. How bad could it be? They had done a number of chest X-rays when you had your bout with pneumonia and the doctors knew you had had lung cancer ten years ago. There shouldn't be any surprises when they looked at your X-rays. Right?

Wrong. Something deep and forbidding inside me, something karmic, removed from my consciousness, already knew that this time "bad" was a different kind of *bad*. Ten years ago, when I thought you were dying, I had asked for just ten more years with you. I should have asked for more.

I told myself to relax, breathe, to loosen my grip on the steering wheel. God wouldn't do this again, no way. We had definitely paid our dues. Neil was too good. Having had his own personal epiphany, he was almost pure. He had made his peace long ago and made reparations for past indiscretions. He was a great father and husband.

A thought popped into my head. Your boss would certainly fire you now, regardless of how good you were at your job. I would have to support us again for a few more weeks. I didn't know how much longer I could do this. What kind of thoughts were these to be having at this time?

My mind drifted in the afternoon sun as I sat in the summer traffic. I remembered a time when we were much younger, when we would go to Gurney's Inn for long weekends, just to get away. We needed to feel the salt air on our faces, the sun on our backs, to swim and fish and eat. You loved to fish and swim. I loved to eat. You taught me how to fish properly and cast like a sailor, not a girl. I remember the beauty of how you swam laps and how people would stand around the pool, watching you. You were always a man of uncommon grace and beauty. You always wanted to teach me things I thought I had no reason to learn. You always strived to make me more independent, as if you knew that our time together was not without end. Regardless, time wove our lives tightly together into a richly textured fabric that now makes looking back a blessing.

There was a succession of ever-worsening phone calls as I sat and cursed, the cell phone in one hand the other rhythmically beating away my nervous energy on the steering wheel. Unable to get to you, I was panicking. I was always better with you by my side, no matter what. You gave me strength and courage when I would otherwise have none. I tried to process the stream of mind-boggling information. Where was your adrenal gland? How big was the mass? Could your brother on Long Island get to the hospital, as I clearly could not? I didn't want you to be alone. Although you did your best to conceal it from me, I heard the crack in your voice. *Please forgive me, I will be there. I'm trying Neil.* Don't panic, we've done this before... remain calm, emotionally neutral. Think, breathe, fix your makeup. Remember, this is the time when your character shows, part of this strength was learned by living with Neil. I said to myself, remember who you are; where you come from, that you are tougher and smarter than they know, don't panic. Just get there! Get to him. He needs you.

I got there eventually—to the wrong hospital. I spent fifteen eternal minutes at the front desk, hovering like a hummingbird with my heart beating wildly until the attendant confirmed you weren't there. When I finally got to the right one, the sun had long set. A tremendous banner hung out front that read "Voted #1 by AARP." I thought to myself, well this looks good. If you're going to have major medical crises, certainly a huge, modern, well-funded hospital is the place to do it.

Four days later we were still waiting for an MRI, although several interns had offered to provide a digital rectal exam in the hallway the very first day. The second day things livened up. Neil's room-mate, an insomniac with a penchant for all-night TV, attempted suicide in the bathroom by cutting his wrists. Luckily, Neil had woken up to pee and saw the blood pooling under the bathroom door. He rang for the nurse, and rang again. Waiting until he could wait no longer, he got himself up, I.V. in tow, and forced the bathroom door open. His roommate fell off the toilet, splattering the pool of his own blood. Eventually, the staff got there and cleaned up. It was the first of many 2:00 a.m. phone calls. The hospital tried to bill us for the door. We were just glad we did not go to the hospital rated #2.

Luckily, four or five days later I was able to get Neil released. Bringing him home was the first of many jubilant trips home from various hospitals. Even at the very end, there was no place more sustaining or significant than home.

Neil and I refused to admit that this was the beginning of the end. In retrospect, I both hate and love those days. I love them because I still had Neil, and we were both too stubborn and proud to sur-render. We both thought that if we pretended things were OK, then somehow they would be. I took a picture of him that first day at home. There was something in his face, something beyond worry. It was a look I couldn't understand, a look that the pho-tographer in me just had to capture and preserve. That photo-graph haunts me still.

Neil knew our remaining time together would be short. We drank Sauvignon Blanc on the deck out back and tried not to think, lost in the sunsets. Our kisses became much more lingering and significant, even as our sex life left us. We often fell asleep in each others arms, sometimes afraid to let go. Our conversations were deep and meaningful. We tried to squeeze a lifetime into a few brief months. We tried to keep the fear at bay. It's a hard concept, dying. But you find that you can love someone so much that in the end, you put aside your own fears. Somehow you know that the only thing you have left to do is to find the strength to let them go.

Neil was Neil, that's why I loved him. Who he was is why I fell in love with him and didn't stop loving him ever, for twenty years, in good times and bad. He had the uncanny ability to make me believe in the impossible time after time. He made me sure that it was perfectly normal to love and marry a man seventeen years my senior. He made me believe that he would beat this cancer again and I believed him, unequivocally. He was graceful and proud. He waited until the day after our wedding anniversary to die. He waited for his son to say goodbye. He held my hand to the very last breath, and I know it was more to calm my fears than his. He waited and suffered until I became, reluctantly, able to let him go.

Neil was good and kind and righteous. I remain a witness to his life and I survive in his place. That's how I think of myself today: as a survivor. It is this thought that sustains me and pushes me on. Always towards life, no matter how difficult that pursuit may at times be. The memory of Neil, his struggles and triumphs lives on through me and the stories we tell of his life.

God Speed, my love, I've got your back. Always.

A Chief Financial Officer by trade, Tracey lives in Northern Westchester County, New York. Writing is a hobby and passion, and she has had several works of poetry published in the recent past.

I Didn't Get the Memo

Karen Laven

No one ever sent me the memo about what to do when you are sandwiched beside your mother in a tiny, pungent doctor's office, waiting to hear why there happened to be a shadow on her X-ray and a liter of fluid in her lungs. There was no note that told me what to say after her longtime physician popped in and informed my sixty-nine year-old mom that the reason for all her complications was that she had lung cancer, complete with a hefty, inoperable tumor inside the left lobe.

The long haired, blonde, blue-eyed doctor informed us that even though mom had quit smoking ten years ago, she now had a specific mumbo-jumbo type of cancer that looked to be Stage IV.

Huh?

I recall asking the woman in white before us what the hell Stage IV meant. She hesitated. I piped in, "Wouldn't Stage I be the worst?"

No? Oh. Nevertheless, isn't there a Stage V for those who are really bad?

We were told that Stage IV covers that dire scenario just fine. I don't remember what I said after that, but I do remember feeling remarkably distant and nauseated. I remember the beauty queen with a stethoscope prescribing Ativan for Mom and handing me a referral for a cancer specialist. What was the point in seeing a specialist if there wasn't anything that could be done? I wanted to ask, but I didn't. I recall wanting to ask the doctor if her mom was alive and well.

That maddeningly sunny September afternoon, as I drove home the person who had raised me, I kept thinking that this wasn't fair—for me. I'd already lost a parent, and right now I desperately wanted my dad. No such luck: he'd died of a heart attack fifteen years earlier.

"I miss your father," Mom said, tears spilling over. I couldn't reply; my throat closed. "I'm so lucky I have you," she added with a smile.

Lucky to have me? The person who has somehow found a way to feel sorry for herself at *your* terminal diagnosis?

That was the beginning of many thoughts and feelings that would humble and sadden me. Mom was smiling. I couldn't smile. I could barely drive. How could she smile? She not only could, she smiled every day throughout the next fourteen months.

I, however, undertook the drama side of it all. When I was apart from Mom, I'm ashamed to say I often cried, screamed and wailed at the unfairness of my life. I had friends and relatives who not only still had their moms around—in great health—but their fathers too. Why did they get to have both their parents while I would soon have neither?

How atrocious was I? Was I secretly wishing that they would lose a parent? Would that make my loss easier? Would that make everything "fair?" My Lord, what was my mother's cancer diagnosis doing to me?

The compassion within me slipped into high gear to help my mother prolong and enjoy what was left of her life. But I was completely spent when out of her sight. I cringe at my selfishness throughout much of Mom's cancer experience. I helped her keep up with shopping and cleaning and took her to her doctor appointments and chemo treatments. I became enraged at my siblings for not pitching in more. I used guilt tactics—whatever I could—to reach them. I wanted someone to help me help Mom. I wanted them to worry about her, wipe her face after she vomited and get angry like I did when she would let herself suffer by not taking her pain pills.

Now that I look back, I think my siblings were afraid to tip the boat. After all, I had everything under control, right? I became very knowledgeable about Mom's treatment and what she needed as far as pills and other cancer-related issues. Believe me, I let my brother and sisters know it.

The truth is, Mom and I had always been close. We did most of our grocery and clothes shopping together. We held word game tournaments. We baked cookies. But I hated when she'd meander into a shoe store—which was a given if there was one within sight. She'd pick up a sandal, a pump and a boot and then ask the salesman if they all came in narrow and I'd stand behind her, tapping my foot impatiently. She also had a way of cajoling me into playing Scrabble with her when I should have been working on my feature story for the paper, and rubbing it in when she won.

As the months edged by, the shopping sessions decreased and then stopped altogether. I was out alone now, picking up her necessities and passing right by the shoe store. Then came the time she could only make it out of the house to go to church... and then not even for that. It was at this point when the Scrabble game started collecting dust.

Finally, when she lay in my son's bedroom, atop a hospice bed, the purple tide creeping within her fingers and toes, she continued to fight and moan in pain. She was given more morphine, and she still had more pain. Finally her breathing liquefied and she called for me from down the hall.

I walked in and stood by her side. I'd think that each breath would be her last, but over and over, another breath followed. Minute after minute, she clutched life and the pain that it contained. I was in agony seeing her agony. She hadn't been cognizant for hours. She took another bubbling breath and then another. I didn't know if she could hear or understand me, but I leaned down and whispered into her ear: "Mom, your pain is killing me."

She then did something that must have taken phenomenal strength. She clenched her mouth shut, refusing to take those breaths that a body automatically clings to, even in the throes of death. Before I could realize what I'd done, she was gone. She had gone to save me more agony.

I think that if I had gotten that memo—the one to tell me what to do to help a loved one through their terminal cancer diagnosis—it would have done me good if it had said, do what's right. Don't ask why others are or aren't doing this, or what's fair. If others want to help you, let them. If they aren't able to, for whatever reason, don't allow this to tarnish your relationship with them or their relationship with the person who has cancer. Be honest about what terminal means. It is excruciating, but don't allow yourself to believe you will have plenty of time later to be a good person. Be as good a person as you can be now. That doesn't mean perfect. It won't happen. Just be your best. That means be there for them.

Yes, you will become agitated and exhausted and frightened, but you will also have the chance to make their days, and what remains of your own life, better. Don't be condescending. Keep humor, compassion and your basic relationship intact. If you don't do this, your conscience will remind you about it over and over until your own time comes to pass.

Shut your mouth and open your heart as you drive them to the shoe store and don't complain about how boring it is and how long they're taking looking for that darn size 7-1/2, narrow loafer.

Above all, play Scrabble every single day and rub it in when you win.

Karen Laven's poetry, articles and essays have appeared in magazines around the country. After seven years writing for a Minnesota newspaper, Karen moved to Kentucky, where she lives with her husband, two sons and their toy poodle.

Easing My Pain

Sandy McPherson Carrubba

If pain were a locomotive moving through one's life, my father was deaf to its clanging bell and skipped around its crushing wheels. An excellent amateur athlete his entire life, he could ignore his frequent injuries and his refusal to acknowledge pain was astounding. Dad always played ice hockey without a helmet. After breaking his thumb playing baseball, he managed to keep bowling by having the hole in his ball drilled wider to fit his swollen finger. One summer, a baseball broke his glasses and cut his eye. Dad just said he was glad he would only have a small scar on his retina.

My father and I did not get on well. Ours had never been a demonstrative family; just as he refused to dwell on pain, Dad was more than reserved in expressing affection and love. He seemed distant and disinterested when I was growing up. We spoke harsh words to one another when I was a teenager, words that lingered long after they were spoken.

So it was unusual when, in the winter of 1975, Dad complained about shoulder pain. Fifty-eight years old at the time, he was past most physically demanding sports but he had kept his energy and never sat still for long. If he wasn't gardening or playing with his young grandchildren, he was working with his saw or metal lathe.

He built model trains and thought up fun games for his grandchildren. He stayed active and did not normally rest during the day.

But during our trips to see him in the summer of 1976 we would find him sitting in his recliner, too tired for his usual pleasures. He finally made a rare visit to our family doctor; the fact that Dad went to a doctor with a complaint made me worry about how serious his ailment could be. But I felt comforted knowing he had sought help. I trusted the doctors to find a solution. Modern medicine would stop that train.

Our doctor could not find the cause of his discomfort or lethargy. He sent Dad to a specialist, who could find nothing suspicious and wanted to prescribe pain pills. Dad refused them and went to another specialist, who was also unable to discover the cause of his complaints. By this time, Dad was frustrated. He had agreed to X-rays and tests, yet he still had no answer, so he stopped going to physicians. Instead, he spent a lot of time sleeping when home from work.

In October, when Dad developed a persistent cough, our doctor suspected pneumonia and sent him to a thoracic specialist. That doctor surprised us with the diagnosis of lung cancer. At last, the train had a name.

By that time, the cancer had advanced so far that Dad was given only six months to a year to live. The news stunned me. I fought for my footing as the world suddenly tipped sideways. I was filled with fear and disbelief. I couldn't help thinking he would have bought himself more time if he hadn't stopped seeing doctors. What if the cancer had been found a year sooner? I prayed to God for a physical healing. Instead, our family received a healing of our souls.

Each week, I took Dad for radiation treatments and watched him decline. His once luxurious brown hair turned grey and fine and fell out. Helpless and agonized, I wanted to help him, to take away his pain just for a day. Fortunately, I had young children and I found distraction from my grief in their youthful excitement and joy. Not able to understand that their beloved "Bop" was very sick, they laughed and played with him in their carefree way. Sometimes the train took a different track—out of sight—and I could join in the play, thoroughly absorbing myself in my children's needs. Halloween that year gave us a chance to be together as a family. We didn't canvass the neighborhood, but went to my Dad's house. Dad was in bed when we arrived, but awoke when he heard our laughter. That day was filled with lots of teasing and fun.

Finally, Dad was hospitalized. His pain had intensified. Coughing spells prevented him from keeping down the paltry amount of food he managed to eat. Fearing he would give up, my mother decided not to tell Dad that his illness was terminal. I disagreed, but abided by her wishes. The pain of our impending separation surrounded my heart. During his hospital stay, I prayed that I could find the strength to tell him that I loved him.

I finally found that strength one day as my mother and I were preparing to leave the hospital. I walked to Dad's bedside, bent down close to his face and whispered "I love you." He seemed startled and pleased by the news. I was so relieved I almost floated out of the hospital. After that, my father and I felt comfortable to simply sit together in silence, holding one another's hand.

One day he said, "I want to know. The doctors won't tell me. Am I going to get better?" My mother began to cry, unable to say the dreaded words. I had to spit them out as if to avoid their bitter taste. "No, Dad, you aren't."

"Oh," he said with his characteristic acceptance, "That's the way the ball bounces."

I left the room to compose myself. When I returned, my mother was sitting on the bed still crying and Dad was rubbing her back, trying to console her. If only we could rub away the cancer as Dad tried to erase Mom's grief. I still see that picture of my parents in my head almost every day and each time I do I experience the same bereft feeling.

That day, at home from the hospital, I got on my hands and knees and scrubbed my kitchen floor. With every swipe of the cloth, I tried to wash away my pain and heartbreak. On other days, I raked leaves or walked our dog or chased her in the yard. Physical activity helped me bear the stress of watching my father so ill.

We were given permission to bring our children to Dad's room for Christmas and New Year's Day. The children sang to Dad as he played with their dolls. He pretended the dolls talked as they "walked" on his bed. Our little girls giggled. Pain was a distant memory for a short time then as we turned our despair into love and laughter.

Nurses told us that after our visits, Dad requested pain medication. He never acted as if he were uncomfortable when we were there. His habit of ignoring pain helped us to get the most from our time with him. I could even imagine that Dad felt better, that his discomfort had abated during our visits. And when I convinced myself of that, I could sleep through the night without disturbing thoughts charging through my brain.

Dad's health insurance paid for six months of hospital care and we had nearly reached that limit. In early March we had him transferred to the local Veteran's Administration Hospital. The week after Dad arrived, his ankles swelled. Still, he never complained when we were with him. Contrasting his newly frail physique with his former athletic one, he pointed to them and quipped, "At least something on me is a decent size." Though Dad acted nonchalant about the swelling, I knew it wasn't a good sign and wondered if his journey was nearing its end.

On the morning of March 13, the nurse called and said, "Your father says you had better come." None of us needed her to explain what that meant.

He took the entire day to die. His strength ebbed so that he could only whisper to us. He was obviously uncomfortable, but totally aware of what was happening. He had become incontinent. Each time he soiled himself, he asked that we call someone to clean him up. It pained me to leave the room each time that happened because I didn't want to give up a minute of the precious time we had left.

Late that evening, the pain in his legs became unbearable. He rubbed them and cried, over and over, "Oh, my legs. My legs." It must have been excruciating, for him to complain in our presence. Watching him was torture for me. We needed to put the brakes on that locomotive. I called the nurse and asked that he be given something for the pain. She argued that it was not yet time; she had to stick to the medication schedule. "What does time matter to someone who has none?" I asked her. She relented. Gradually the medication took effect and Dad drifted to sleep.

The pauses in his breathing became longer and longer. Finally his breathing stopped and he looked peaceful. I felt a kind of peace in the room. Gone was the tension caused by his pain.

"Oh, how beautiful," my mother said over and over. Dad appeared relaxed and looked truly beautiful. Knowing Dad had gone to a place where there is no pain helped some.

My father suffered throughout the five and a half months of his final illness, but he tried his best to hide his intense pain from us. His final gift was his lucidity on his last day. But, I don't know if I could have remained strong enough to accompany him on his journey if we hadn't finally reconciled. Having spoken those words of love at his bedside made sharing that long train ride bearable.

A graduate of the State University of New York at Oswego, Sandy's writing career spans fifty years. A married mother of two, she is active in church and environmental causes.

Continued from page (212)

Hospice Care

In dealing with the final course of the disease, your medical team will eventually talk to you about hospice. That word, when first mentioned sometimes means the final step before death. However, hospice has evolved into an extension of your physician's treatment to provide the most sophisticated and aggressive therapies available to almost eliminate most of the troublesome symptoms that lung cancer can cause in its later stages. Hospice does not always mean the end of life. The intense treatment given to relieve physical symptoms and psychological, emotional and spiritual distress improves the physical and the emotional state of the patient. At times, the improvement may be enough to allow the patient to come off the program for an additional attempt at chemotherapy. If such an attempt is successful, the patient may not need to use the resources of hospice for long. If the new attempt at treatment is unsuccessful, the patient can come back to hospice. There have been some cases, although rare, in which a patient's terminal illness was so improved that she was able to enter into a prolonged period of stability.

The hospice team usually includes highly trained palliative care nurses, social workers for family counseling, a volunteer companion program, a spiritual worker, a bereavement specialist and the hospice team's palliative care medical director. This team will give the patient and family the most advanced care. 24-hour live on-call staff, including physician backup is always available, preventing trips to the emergency room and admissions to the hospital. If a patient must be hospitalized because of an especially severe symptom or problem, most hospices have specially designed inpatient units with a home-like environment to deliver the necessary medical care. Hospice will provide this therapy and support in an atmosphere of hope where the patient feels that an entire medical team is still working for him or her with only one purpose, to make their remaining life as fruitful, productive and comfortable as possible. There is simply no better substitute for care of the patient in the last stages of lung cancer.

Continued on page (250)

Destination Unknown
Felicia Monticelli

One March morning, my husband called me from work to tell me that Dana Reeve, the wife of actor Christopher Reeve, had passed away.

The previous August, when she was diagnosed with lung cancer, I was sitting in a hospital bed after a summer of dealing with an increasingly bad cough. At first I was told I had bronchitis and later, pneumonia. Because I was only thirty-five and a nonsmoker, it never crossed my family doctor's mind that I might have cancer. The average age of a person diagnosed with lung cancer is seventy-one.

A lung specialist put me in the hospital to run a multitude of tests and isolate me for possible TB. Just before being admitted I called my husband, who was in Italy for a cousin's wedding. In my extreme way, I joked, "Watch, you'll come home and I'll have lung cancer." When my husband did get back to the States, he was minutes too late to be by my side for the diagnosis.

Through the last six months of chemotherapy, medications, and scans, Dana Reeve has been on my mind. She was one of my beacons to help give me hope. This morning as I ate breakfast, the news of her death weighed on me. My sister (who came to live with me and help care for my daughter this year) reminded me that I have made tremendous progress. I told her, "I guess I am going to have to be my own poster child now."

Trying to keep upbeat yet be realistic about this disease is my greatest challenge. The statistics for survival are dismal. Lung cancer usually doesn't present symptoms until the late stages and often not until it has metastasized. This is the case for me.

In November, as I started to feel better, my situation really hit me. The advice my oncologist gave was to do all my planning for death and then, "put it all in a pretty pink box and live." In planning for death, he was of course thinking of a will and other more official matters. For the mother of a four-year-old, planning for death takes on a different urgency and becomes an unending project to pass on some kind of legacy. So my box keeps filling. In fact, it has become several real boxes. On days when I have some energy, I do what I can. I've organized twenty-two years of journals that will give my daughter some picture of me throughout my life. I've made videos of us reading books and playing. I've written a coming-of-age letter to her and placed it in a box with some of my favorite books. My current journal is being filled with stories I would have told her about my own life as she was growing up. And while all these things don't equal what I could give her as a living mother, I feel I am making use of what life has brought my way. When I do dare to hope for the future, I imagine myself by her side as she opens these little treasures, put away long ago.

Cancer has made painfully clear how solid my picture of the future had been. Now I can see ahead only as far as my next scan. I balance hope with what needs to be done if I don't make it. One of my daily practices before becoming ill was to open the Tao Te Ching and meditate on whichever passage I found. The day after my diagnosis I opened to verse number 59, and this portion stood out for me. It helped me when I was very ill and continues to help me deal with low energy days:

The mark of a moderate [woman]

Is freedom from [her] own ideas.

Tolerant like the sky,

All pervading like sunlight,

Firm like a mountain,

Supple like a tree in the wind,

[She] has no destination in view,

And makes use of anything life happens to bring [her] way.

Nothing is impossible for [her]

Because [she] has let go.*

Hailing from central New York, Felicia became Writing Center Manager at Frederick Community College in Frederick, MD in 2000. Since her medical leave in August 2005 she has remained an avid reader, journal writer, and artist.

*Stephen Mitchell trans. Harper Perennial, 1992.

Taking Care
Joann Price

Sometimes I wonder what happened to my life. It moved along bit by bit, baffling me, throwing me into a world of fatigue, worry and unease. That was the past. I ask, what about right now?

My constant concern now is about my aging and very sick father. He didn't ask for this insidious cancer. He wonders why me, why now? He wonders if the treatment is worth it, yet he isn't capable of stopping the process, because he is weak in mind and spirit. I see it in his eyes sometimes, the glazed look as someone speaks to him. He doesn't answer or he gazes down and finally says something that has little to do with the question.

How can I help him? Will my care matter? Will it make a difference? Am I doing enough? I wonder about my life too. I know it's not about me; it's about him and my duty as a daughter. It is about my responsibility to the other members of my family. Is it up to me to care for him so he lives longer and they can see him, talk to him? I hang onto the fact that we are all aging and have families of our own. We know that our one surviving parent is still alive to remind us of our childhood and what love means.

I cannot take my mother's place nor replace what my father lost when she died of lung cancer. Does he think about the care he tried to give her years ago? Does he remember what it was like to hop up every few minutes to provide something, even if it's just a smile or a slight touch on the forearm? Does he remember the worry when the discomfort is so plainly seen, or the pain becomes something that can't be managed any longer? Maybe he has wiped most of those memories from his mind. Who can blame him?

What about him? What will the next weeks and months hold? Will we, a year from now, look back and take a deep breath and remember one more time that we are glad it is over? Will it be one more time, thank God, that he is playing golf and going out to dinner? Will I, weeks and months from now, be in the same place or in another place that I don't understand or wish for? Only God knows because it is obviously His plan.

I put my hands to my forehead and rub and rub. I rub my upper arms and shoulders, willing the aches to go away. I listen to him cough. I listen to his soft footsteps as he makes his way from the living room to the kitchen and carefully down the stairs. He isn't as sure-footed as he wants to be and I wait, holding my breath until he settles down again. When I wake in the morning I must bound from bed, in case he needs me and doesn't want to disturb my own rest. I listen to the toilet flush, knowing he has made his way to the toilet on the other side of his room, and glad that there is still a normal human act, and I breathe out again.

There is indignity to all this. There is some embarrassment to this care giving, an embarrassment between a father and daughter. What will I have to do for him yet, to make it easier, swallowing the difficulty of it all for both of us, and plunging forward to do what must be done? I don't want to go there. But it isn't about me.

Before I get out of bed and open the bedroom door to face the morning, I tell myself over and over that he has the hard part. I've closed the door to have peace, even for a few minutes. I close the door to have my life back, even for a while.

I'm not usually one to get teary-eyed. Lately though, that is exactly what I've been doing. I've been crying at night, as silently as I can. I've cried in the shower. I've cried as I put laundry in the washer and dryer. It seems so overwhelming most of the time that it is easy to lose control as I watch him get weaker. I remind myself that selfishness is unbecoming in a mature woman. After all, when I was ill my parents took care of me. But should my life be turned upside down? Should everyone's life, but his and mine, go on, with only casual, occasional reminders of his plight? Why should my life be the one that is not the same? But those thoughts are just poor me thoughts, and I've no right to have them.

I'm afraid for him; I'm afraid he will suffer, and I will have to watch him, care for him, do what must be done, the most that can be done to help him not suffer. Fear is such a strong emotion, and I know he is afraid. If I am to help him with that fear, am I allowed to have fears of my own?

Early this morning I went for a long walk. I looked up at the vast blue sky and I tried to take deep breaths as I took my steps. I tried so hard to see the beauty, to bring the fresh air into my lungs, to ask God for His blessings, for patience, for forgiveness and mercy. Autumn leaves gently floated onto the street and onto the still green lawns. I relished the walk. I wanted to clear my head. I didn't want to return home. But I had to. And when I stepped through the back door, I mouthed the words, "Is he up yet?" And my dear mate, who had already made the coffee and provided the multitude of prescribed medications, nodded yes, and by the look on his face, I knew that Dad didn't feel well. My mate's looks warned me to steel myself, to prepare myself, to shed the light of a beautiful autumn morning and brace myself for another trying day. I stepped into the kitchen and Dad, sitting at the kitchen table, the newspaper sports section in front of him, said he didn't feel at all well.

Life has not been kind to my father. Sometimes he smiles and tells stories, stories I've heard many times before, and sometimes stories that are new and make me smile. What a privilege it is to listen. What a gift to be there, listening.

Life is often difficult. Everyone knows this. Everyone knows that life is full of joys, sadness and frustrations. Life comes with love and hate. It comes with resentments, dangers, highs and lows. It happens to every one of us, and it isn't what happens so much as what follows that really matters. In life, both joy and sadness change the heart. I think about its shape. Is it round and smooth, or are the edges ragged, damaged? Do my tears change the shape of my heart and does my smile, even my laughter, heal it? I wonder and then I wonder some more!

Sometime, hours, days, months from now, I will look back on this time and hopefully I will wonder how I did it all, and maybe feel proud of these long, difficult days. I hope that I will look back and think about it with a strong faith, not one that is weak, dispirited. I hope I will feel relief with deep breaths, rather than shoulders that sag, or even shake, with my moaning. Yes, relief, liberation, a hope for life's relief, certainly for him, and for me. I am left to *wonder and wonder some more!*

The author is a college English teacher, writer, reader, and a writing coach. Married for 30 years and a mother and grandmother, she hopes to move to the northwest coast where she can write and read by the sea.

Crossing Borders
Dee Redfearn

Pearl, a spirited Texas blonde, is the Florence Nightingale of the Puerto Aventura community, always helping someone in need. The night before Ronn and I left our Yucatan condo to return to Washington, D.C., Pearl appeared at our door with a platter of cannabis cookies—for the pain between my husband's shoulder blades, she said. Ronn and I exchanged smiles as we silently contemplated the medicinal qualities of Pearl's offering.

Ronn had been diagnosed with cancer six months before. Even without hair and thinner than usual, at sixty-seven he had retained his Steve McQueenish rugged-guy good looks. As we studied Pearl's cookies, I knew his suffering was more from the thought of leaving these people and this place than from the constant pain. One local offered a juice program she had learned in Oaxaca; another a Reiki session; another, medicinal massage learned in Thailand. Each good intention brought its own healing powers— kindness and humor to sustain us.

These local offerings were a far cry from the latest treatments and clinical trials my husband had received at Johns Hopkins Medical Center in Baltimore. Some weeks before we left Puerto Aventura, Ronn, who, unlike me, thought most traditional methods bogus, relented and let me drive him to Dr. Carmen, an acupuncturist.

She, like the natives and our friend Pearl, resorted to alternative methods.

Dr. Carmen's office was in her home built on stilts under a huge, Mayan-inspired, palm leaf *palapal* roof. The doctor answered the door wearing a medical smock that had once been white; silver threads streaked hair that had once been black. Her strong handshake rallied our confidence. To reach her office, we followed a stone path set in a bed of flowers. A staircase in the middle of the main room led to a loft where she obviously slept, a heap of medical books for her pillow. We could only guess, or hope rather, that she had read them. Strands of multicolored crystal beads hung floor to ceiling, dividing us from the treatment room. I tugged on Ronn's shirt sleeve and pointed to a diploma that hung on the wall. A medical degree?

I explained my husband's condition. Although I did not have the Spanish vocabulary to explain non-small cell lung cancer, I struggled through. She nodded, peering over her dark rimmed glasses. I stayed to watch the doctor open a new packet of needles and watched Ronn remove his shirt and lie face down on the table. "I can help," I heard Dr. Carmen say as I fumbled through the bead curtain and escaped to the waiting room.

Time, which may have been only a brief moment, passed at a *mañana* pace. Finally I heard a resounding, "Dee. Where the hell are you?"

"I'm here." I leapt from my chair. "Are you in pain?"

"I feel like a goddamn pincushion."

I thanked Dr. Carmen and paid for Ronn's release with one hundred and fifty pesos, the equivalent of fifteen U.S.dollars, and left. On the road, Ronn and I exchanged glances as we did after so many years together, communicating in silence.

The next morning Ronn announced that he wanted to go back to Hopkins. I realized that, by increments, it had become more diffi-

THE HEALING PROJECT 241 VOICES OF LUNG CANCER

cult for him to walk—not because his motor skills were affected, but because the pain between his shoulder blades had brought him to conclude, "This ain't living."

I booked our flight, made arrangements for a car to pick us up and packed an overnight bag (medical records, drugs, ice pack and toothbrush, nothing more.) Working our way through the airport lines was less of a challenge than coaxing my tall, proud, Texas husband to sit in a wheel chair. Amazed at how water parts to let a wheel chair pass, I wheeled Ronn past security to the nearest coffee stand and left him to read the first U.S. newspaper he had seen in three weeks. I hadn't gotten far when the announcement came over a loudspeaker. "United Flight 2242 to Philadelphia has been canceled."

"No *problema*," the ticket agent explained, holding hands palms-out like a traffic cop. "We have free hotel, free drinks, and free food for everyone." He was the only one smiling.

"For how long?" I projected over the crowd.

"*¿Quién sabe?* For as long as it takes." He smiled and shrugged.

"No. You don't understand. *Es emergencia.* There are several here."

"*¿Es emergencia?*" he repeated.

"*Sí, emergencia. Emergencia urgente.*" I explained that our daughter was picking us up in Philly to drive my husband directly to the hospital cancer center.

"Ahhh, give me your boarding pass. Come back in half an hour."

I smiled as naturally as I could and joined Ronn for coffee. Ten minutes before our planned departure, I excused myself and went in search of the ticket agent. He avoided my glance and spoke just past my shoulder to a dozen hands shaking tickets in his face. One nonchalant glance down, index finger to lip, he returned my boarding passes along with a note. Checking over my shoulder, as if something illicit had just transpired, I hid behind a pillar and unfolded the note: "See Jorge at gate seven."

I slipped the secret code in my purse—*número siete*, Jorge. Yes!

At Gate Seven we had to draw a number and stand in line, but finally an official wheeled Ronn aboard with me following. "We made it," I whispered in Ronn's ear; he patted my wrist.

"Welcome aboard first class." A cute stewardess flashed a Trident smile. First class? *Too good to be true*, I thought. And it was.

"Where are we headed?" Ronn asked.

"Charleston."

Not to worry, she assured us after I explained our destination and planned ETA. Sure, you can make a connection. Well, no, not Philly or Baltimore, but D.C. When we landed, it was almost midnight. An angel appeared wearing a red cap. No wings, but his warm smile more than made up for Washington's forty-degree weather for a couple still dressed for the Yucatan. He had a wheel chair waiting at the door of the plane and hailed a cab for us.

By the following week, Ronn was admitted to the intensive care unit, not in Baltimore, but at the Lombardi Cancer Center at Georgetown Hospital in D.C. There he fought his last good fight. Eight days later, without suffering and surrounded by family, he peacefully surrendered.

It took me two months to settle affairs and emotions and carry out Ronn's wishes. I boarded United, alone this time, carrying a handsomely carved cherry wood box containing Ronn's ashes. I was taking my husband back to his beloved Yucatan. I came prepared for anything that could possibly go wrong. I had called the airline ahead of time, brought a briefcase of documents (death certificate, marriage certificate, cremation permit, and both our passports), just in case. Sitting alone aboard the 747, I patted the top of the box. "We made it," I whispered.

Before I arrived at our home, Daniel, the groundskeeper, had opened the sliding doors that led out to the balcony. The night was black, as only Yucatan skies can be. The only light reflected from the boats below. I put the cherry wood box on a rough wood table in the middle of the room and made my way to the kitchen. The freezer door made a sucking sound when I pulled it open and a puff of cold fog slapped my face. The cannabis cookies were gone. Either the housekeeper had done her job well or she and Pearl had made off with the goods. So I sat with the box containing Ronn's mortal remains and spoke to his spirit about tomorrow and the last leg of his journey.

"Tomorrow I will dress in white pants made from light cotton weave loose enough to sieve wind, and a white shirt woven by the Zapotecs, and rope sandals from Xel Ha, and a wide-brim straw hat and dark glasses, befitting a widow. I will carry you in a basket of flowers that our grandsons will have picked. Our daughters, Ashley and Victoria, and our grown sons, Todd and Tim, will follow the caravan of mourners. And Philippe, a local boat boy, will have a skiff large enough for the family and a good friend to board. Sebastian, three years old now, will sit at the bow of the boat and toss a trail of flowers over the water where we will launch you on your journey. And Sergio, the gypsy from San Miguel who wears shells around his ankle that clatter with each strum of his guitar, will play soft chords. And his friend, José, a Mayan flautist, will play primitive tones on his pan-flute that will carry across the ocean."

And the universe will be at peace.

The next day, a persimmon globe sun made its slow descent into the horizon. I couldn't have asked for more colorful serenity, or purer beauty. There, near a dock of pitted stone where waves had lapped for a thousand years, we gathered to speak last thoughts of our friend, the sailor, the seeker, the *bon vivant*, while José's pan-flute sent ripples across the ocean for miles and miles and miles.

The author is a graduate of the Johns Hopkins Advanced Academic Program in fiction writing where she was nominated for "Best New Voices" 2003 and 2004. She is a recent finalist for New Letter's fiction award. A former educator, she has worked with the mentally challenged at the Children's Development in Dallas. She now resides in Washington D.C. and divides her time between there and the Yucatan peninsula.

I Can Find You
in the Wind

Alicia Gregory

The day my mother died I was sixteen going on five going on twenty-three. Eating peanut butter and jelly for the first time in so many years, I stared out the dining room window at a cold December morning. Death was swimming through the rooms, making me uncomfortable in my own home. I was like a child on her first day of school, tentative and nervous over the idea of leaving her mother for a day. Ten years later, I had regressed to childhood, only now I was nervous about my mother leaving me.

I watched her so closely that morning, afraid that each shallow breath was her last. I didn't think I would be ready. *Not right now*, I thought. *Please, not now.* Every minute I worked on preparing myself for The Moment, as if it were something that could be scripted, even planned for. The moment when she would let go and I would automatically be initiated into the exclusive group of motherless daughters. Those girls people would worry about, pity, who would be more apt to veer off track. Those girls who would give their traumatized fathers heart attacks, the ones who would sit defiantly in family therapy, refusing any exchange of words. You know: the bitter ones. I already loathed the stereotype that was to come with my loss.

I worked on being normal, accepting, understanding. I wanted to take the situation for what it was worth, extract wisdom, maybe a larger understanding of life... I wanted to be brave, strong and certainly not needy. Yet, as normally as I tried to function, it was already happening. The females in the family extending themselves, mothers of friends sending food, volunteering to cook dinner, clean the house. Some established themselves as therapists, there if I "ever needed to talk." Many offered me a place to sleep, like I did not have a room, or a home, or a bed of my own. Did they think the cancer ate my house too?

Though it had been turned into a mini-hospital, allowing my mother the comfort and decency of dying in her own home, and though the faces of hospice nurses were as frequent as that of my tired father, I did not feel the need to escape the draining environment even if it was heavy with impending doom and naïve hope for a turnaround, a miracle. I wanted to be right there with my mother, loving her every minute of every day she had left. Except my love for her was not enough, I felt. I wanted to melt into her, become one of her long eyelashes, wrap myself around her heart. This way, I could be with her always. This way, she would be aware of my devotion.

We would never have any closure. The word "cancer" had never been mentioned between us. There had only been sad smiles in the small moments of minimal clarity we were allotted, the tiny moments when she would break through the haze of morphine and we would again be on the same wave. Her sad smiles were apologetic. *I'm sorry I'm leaving you.* They were painful. *So this is the way it is ending?*

Our only conversations were brief and small before she drifted back off into a dreamy fog. What do you say when your time is so limited? How can you possibly express the storm of emotion that churns your insides every day and night—your body trying to come to terms with the impending separation? All I could so eloquently muster was, "I'm sorry. I'm so sorry." In her times of clarity, she would try to comfort me, but her sadness and disappointment were too great to hide. I wanted her to survive so we could laugh about the absurdness of her illness later, write a book like we had vaguely planned, and come out of this hell so much stronger. Many times, just as I was ready to tell her this, I would see her slip back under the morphine. She'd smile and tell me to look at the roses that were growing over the bed. At least her delusions were beautiful.

In the beginning there was so much hope, so many possibilities. I would write to her on post-it notes while she slept in the hospital, never fully able to express how much I wanted to give her the entire world. As if there was some gift monumental enough to make up for the hell that she was experiencing. When did reality set in? The tight feeling of knowing that she was losing the battle, quickly and harshly.

Oh, the knowing. The knowing fashions itself like an uneasiness in the air as it is recognized in looks and glances, or sometimes discovered in the lack of looks and glances. I found that sometimes people would not look at me. The nurses because they felt bad, they knew what was coming. My father, because in me he saw my mother, I was a reminder of what was.

The day my mother died the air hung heavy, moist and grey, nature wept for her. I held her hand and watched her so intensely, watching her breathing fade to something so light that I had convinced myself several times she had left us before it really happened. She went silently and quickly, which, I was told, is rare. Apparently, death at home usually isn't as peaceful as one would think. The nurse told us we were lucky; I heard this as unnecessary detail.

I sat with my mother long after she had gone, memorizing the shape of her face and feeling the warmth of her chest. Essentially, I was holding onto her shell, as if it meant something, as if she were somewhere buried deep down inside, hiding, taking a rest.

Now, almost five years later, five years older, and five years further away from that defining time of my life, the death of my mother has changed everything. It is the singular catalyst that sent me on the road to incredible growth, a complete redefinition of the individual that I was and am. I have yet to experience another moment that was so utterly diminishing, another situation to make me feel as small as dust, as insignificant as a stain on the sidewalk. To be so close to such a mammoth force as death is humbling; to realize that the working of nature is so above us is astounding.

My acceptance of my mother's death came slowly, as I found myself having to give way to the higher force that seemed to rule that endless time, a time of surrendering any power I thought I had, of giving up and accepting defeat. A cluster of multiplying toxic cells had tricked doctors, had put a hole in my family, and had eventually won. Even after life began moving again, even after the hell had passed, I learned what it was to be small, truly, insignificantly small. And yet still, I was able to extract from the dismal experience views on life that can't fully be understood until you have witnessed the power of death.

I started to own the situation, become territorial even. Yes, millions of people lose loved ones to cancer, yet it is never in the same way. My mother had a tumor in her leg so large that it ate away her hip bone and she was bedridden for the better part of four months. She went into a coma on her birthday and almost died. The cancer traveled to her stomach and blocked her digestion so she started throwing up black bile. The details are hellish, the situation a nightmare. Even with all of my newfound wisdom, I became defensive when others would say they knew what I had been through. They didn't. They hadn't seen what I had seen, just as I hadn't seen what they had. My grief was my own and I did not want anyone else trying to touch it.

I fashioned ideas from Whitman to my situation: "All goes onward and outward—nothing collapses." My eyes were widened to a whole new side of things that I had previously been unaware of. That is, I need not weep at my mother's grave, for she is everywhere, in everything. I can find her in the wind; she is the sand that sifts between my toes, the fresh cut grass that tickles my fingers. My mother is a pastel sunrise and the rainbow after a storm. This is where I find my comfort, knowing that in death one becomes part of nature. Now, when I find myself missing my mother, I know I only have to look to the wind.

Alicia Gregory is a student at Hobart and William Smith Colleges in Geneva, NY. She is a native of Southern New Jersey.

Continued from page (230)

Never Lose Hope

I have given you a plan to allow you to get the most out of the healthcare system and maximize the benefits of treatment. Hopefully, this information will increase the odds of a successful outcome in your fight. The important thing is to never lose hope; to maintain the belief that you will beat this illness, to ask questions constantly and to stay informed. Be aggressive in getting what you need to get out of the healthcare system. But most important of all, be positive and determined about your illness, its treatment, your doctors and the outcome. Having a positive attitude, questioning your doctors, getting second opinions and pushing, pushing, pushing can and has often meant the difference between life and death.

Afterword

Into The Future

Michael Vincent Smith, M.D.

This book is very special. It is a family album of sorts. Lung cancer has turned people with nothing in common into brothers and
sisters, uncles, aunts, and cousins. Those who have lung cancer
and those of us who love and care for them are inextricably bound
together. This wonderful collection of stories shares the highs and
lows, the tragedies and triumphs, the despair and the dreams of an
increasingly vocal group of individuals linked by our mutual dis-
dain for this disease. As the son of a lung cancer victim, a practic-
ing thoracic surgeon and a clinical researcher, I was honored when
asked to write the final chapter in this journal. And while the
recurring theme of the preceding stories is one of reflection, I take
this opportunity to look forward, to the future of the diagnosis of
and treatment for this disease. I believe it is a future filled with
hope. While it is always risky to speculate on what tomorrow may
bring, let me suggest what the next 20 years may hold.

Early Detection

CT Scanning

Lung cancer is difficult to detect in its early stages, when therapeutic intervention can make a positive difference, because symptoms usually do not appear until the disease is well advanced. As a result, today between 70%–80% of all lung cancers are diagnosed in the advanced stages (III-IV), resulting in an average five-year survival rate of only 15%. Both chest X-rays and the far more advanced low dose computerized tomography (*CT scan*) have been used with some success in detecting lung cancer earlier; however, with both there is a high incidence of false positive test results and the attendant risk of unnecessary invasive diagnostic procedures and treatments.

The success of CT scanning in detecting early stage cancer is a function of the scanning resolution of the detectors (cameras) used to capture the images and of the medical profession's ability to read and understand the images captured. The more detectors used, the greater the resolution and the greater likelihood that tumors will be found in their early stages. A Japanese company has recently developed a CT scanner with 256 detectors, 8 times the number of detectors in many units still in use. By 2015, the increased resolution and the volume of information obtained from more sophisticated imaging devices will require a level of data collection and analysis beyond our present abilities. But these advances will eventually allow physicians to calculate the growth patterns of tiny nodules in the lung long before metastasis is likely to have occurred. By 2025, the early detection of lung cancer will be the accepted standard of care. The number of lung cancers found in the later stages will fall dramatically and the average five-year survival rate for the disease will climb to about 80%.

Serum and Protein Markers

Imaging technologies will have a dramatic effect on lung cancer mortality and morbidity, but their impact will pale in comparison to the opportunities presented by the identification of biologic markers for lung cancer. *Serum* or *tumor markers* are substances produced by tumor cells that can be found in the blood, the urine, in the tumor tissue or other tissues. Researchers have identified a number of substances that seem to be expressed when some types of cancers are present and that may be used to screen for and detect cancer, determine the stage of the disease and plan appropriate therapy. There has also been some excitement in the area of *proteomics*, the identification and study of human proteins. Several laboratories have analyzed tumor tissue from patients with lung cancer and have discovered protein patterns that could discriminate diseased from healthy tissue and eventually lead to improved screening and early diagnosis.

But the promise of a reliable and widely applicable blood test or protein marker to detect lung cancer in the earliest stages has yet to be fulfilled. Much of the problem lies in the fact that we currently lack the resources and processes to collect and genetically analyze the hundreds of thousands of lung cancer tissue specimens harvested annually worldwide. By 2010, the scientific community will have educated medical practitioners sufficiently or will have pushed policymakers for regulations to support the collection of these specimens. By 2020, biological markers will be a reality and will most likely find early adoption for use with environmentally at-risk patients. Genetic profile analysis will become available by 2025, as we conquer the last frontier of early detection, the genetically predisposed (at-risk) individual.

Diagnosis

While computerized tomography and positron emission tomography are essential tools in lung cancer diagnosis and staging today, their role will diminish as more cancers are detected earlier. This is because metastasis is less likely to occur if the lung cancer is detected early. By 2025, surgical biopsy will give way to less invasive techniques. As technology advances, analysis of the biochemical profiles of tissue will become the standard. Thus, "molecular confirmation" will replace the assessment of cells under a microscope.

Treatment

Chemotherapy

Chemoprevention in lung cancer has been a topic of research for years. However, with a large percentage of cancers being diagnosed only when the disease is already advanced, the only practical "prevention" to date has been chemotherapy given to the previously treated, at-risk-for-recurrence group. However, the ability to identify genetically at-risk individuals and to arrest the progression of abnormal cells to full blown malignancy is likely to become commonplace by 2015. In the same way we now pharmacologically manage diabetes mellitus, hypertension, and human immune deficiency, we will see a group of people controlling their cancer.

The hallmark of care for advanced lung cancer today is based on chemotherapy with or without adjuvant radiation therapy. Only about 20% of patients receiving the most effective chemotherapies in use today will show any response. As a result, the median survival rate for such patients is only 8 months. This unacceptable result is about to be changed drastically by new pharmacologic agents that offer significant new hope to the victims of advanced cancer.

The current drugs generically known as *chemotherapy* or *cytotoxic* (cell destroying) therapy kill cancer cells by directly attacking the process of cell division, destroying the ability of the cancer cell to make new, functioning DNA, RNA and the proteins needed for cellular growth. These drugs block the replication of DNA that is necessary for cell division, or alter cell DNA and cause it to produce faulty RNA, which in turn leads to dysfunctional protein production that disrupts the metabolism of the cell, causing cancer cell death. Unfortunately, these medications are only crudely selective for cancer cells: normal cells are also destroyed by these drugs, which leads to the extensive side effects that make chemotherapy such a dreaded treatment option.

A host of revolutionary new treatments for advanced lung cancer are or will soon be in use. These treatments attack the disease in one of three new, safer and more effective ways. The first of this powerful triumvirate are the *angiogenesis inhibitors*, such as the drug Avastin®. Already used for the treatment of colon cancer with excellent therapeutic results, it has, at the time of this writing, just been approved for use against advanced lung cancer. Representing the vanguard of a whole family of blood vessel development inhibitors that will make their appearance in the next decade, these drugs prevent tiny tumors from developing the blood vessel network they need in order to allow the tumor to grow and spread throughout the body.

The second are the *tyrosine kinase inhibitors*, the so-called "targeting drugs" that interfere with the functioning of a specific growth regulating protein, epidermal growth factor receptor (EGFR), which helps cancer cells divide. Examples of such drugs available today are Iressa® and the even more advanced Tarceva®. These medications are much more specific in their attack on lung cancer cells, thereby reducing the collateral destruction of healthy cells and the dangerous and uncomfortable side effects caused by traditional chemotherapy. As an added benefit, these "targeted therapies" are taken orally, eliminating the complex and prolonged injections and infusions that characterize many of the current treatments.

Finally, the third weapon in the arsenal—*monoclonal antibodies*—when used in tandem with these other drugs, will track down and destroy cancer cells that might survive the angiogenesis inhibitor drugs or that find a way around the metabolic obstacle to growth offered by the "targeting" tyrosine kinase inhibitors. These antibody proteins attach themselves to proteins found on the surface of lung cancer cells and carry with them packets of "poison" in the form of radioactive isotopes or biological toxins that deliver their deadly payload directly to the cancer cells. Normal, healthy cells are spared from destruction, since the healthy cells do not have the proteins found on cancer cells that allow the antibodies to attach to them. These agents have already been very successful in treating lymph gland and breast cancers, and will become a common treatment for lung cancer within the next decade. Moreover, not only will these drugs destroy the cancerous survivors of the other two therapies discussed above, they will do the same to cells resistant to traditional chemotherapy, which will continue to play a role in the treatment of advanced lung cancer into the foreseeable future.

Together with advanced genetic analysis capability, the targeted drug therapies (the so called "*designer-gene*" therapies) will allow customized agents to be developed quickly to improve the success rate of treatment. There will not be just a few targeted therapies, such as the tyrosine kinase or angiogenesis inhibitors. Rather, for patients whose lung cancer was not prevented from occurring, the year 2025 will offer individualized therapy with a huge roster of agents specifically matched to the genetic makeup of their tumors.

Immunotherapy

Stimulation of the patient's immune system has been best used as a means to combat cancer. Given our current knowledge of the importance of immune surveillance in cancer prevention, it is logical to expect continued investigation and advances in this area. Immunotherapeutic agents that strengthen the body's own natural disease-fighting mechanisms will be used in 2025 not only to augment targeted therapy, but also to amplify the response of the immune system to any early re-occurrence of the tumor. New episodes of the disease will be stopped in their tracks before becoming a clinical problem to the patient.

Best Practices

Multidisciplinary care clinics are only now becoming a routine part of the management of lung cancer. The present focus is on participation by thoracic surgeons, medical oncologists and radiation oncologists, supported by nurses and patient advocates. As molecular evaluation, genetic counseling and preventive management become standards of cancer care, the composition of the multidisciplinary team is likely to change. By 2025, the infrequent identification of later-stage lung cancers will make surgical intervention uncommon. As paradoxical as this may sound coming from a surgeon, I welcome the coming of this day.

If the vision I have shared with you seems hard to imagine, consider the following. The first antibiotic was discovered only 78 years ago; prior to that time, death from a simple infection was a common occurrence. Fifty-five years ago, the only computer available occupied an entire room and required 120 seconds to perform a simple addition of two numbers. Seventeen years ago, the standard gallbladder operation was an open procedure with a four day hospitalization; presently the procedure is done on an outpatient basis through a few small holes in the abdomen with an inserted endoscope. Fifteen years ago, there was no world wide web.

It seems only fitting to close with the lyrics from this popular song performed by Fleetwood Mac:

Why not think about times to come,
And not about the things that you've done,
If your life was bad to you,
Just think what tomorrow will do.

Don't stop, thinking about tomorrow,
Don't stop, it'll soon be here,
It'll be, better than before,
Yesterday's gone, yesterday's gone.

Dr. Smith is the Vice-Chairman of the Department of Surgery, Chief of Cardiovascular and Thoracic Surgery and Medical Director of Oncology of the Atlanta Medical Center located in Atlanta Georgia. He is an Associate Adjunct Professor of the Department of Surgery of the Medical College of Georgia; President of the Board of Trustees, Georgia Institute for Lung Cancer Research, Inc.; an Alley-Sheridan Fellow of the Harvard University, Division of Health and Policy Research and Education and a Fellow of the American College of Chest Physicians, the American College of Cardiology and the American College of Surgeons.

Send Us Your Story

Do you have a story to tell? LaChance Publishing and The Healing Project publish four books a year of stories written by people like you. Have you or those you know been touched by life threatening illness or chronic disease? Your story can give comfort, courage and strength to others who are going through what you have already faced.

Your story should be no less than 500 words and no more than 2,000 words. You can write about yourself or someone you know. Your story must inform, inspire, or teach others: tell the story of how you or someone you know faced adversity; what you learned that would be important for others to know; how dealing with the disease strengthened or clarified your relationships or inspired positive changes in your life.

The easiest way to submit your story is to visit The Healing Project website at www.thehealingproject.com or the LaChance Publishing website at www.lachancepublishing.com. There you will find guidelines for submitting your story online, or you may write to us at submissions@lachancepublishing.com. We look forward to reading your story!

Resources

On the following pages you will find information on some of the foremost organizations in the country focused on lung cancer care, research and education and including information on organizations written about by the authors of the essays found in this book.

American Association for Cancer Research
615 Chestnut Street, 17th Floor
Philadelphia, PA 19106
Phone: (215) 440-9300
http://www.aacr.org

The oldest and largest scientific organization in the world focused on innovative cancer research.

American Cancer Society
Phone: (800) ACS-2345
http://www.cancer.org

Learn about cancer and find local support groups throughout the United States

American Institute for Cancer Research
1759 R Street NW
Washington, D.C. 20009
Phone: (202) 328-7744
http://www.aicr.org

Focuses on the nutrition, diet education and research on cancer treatment and prevention.

American Lung Association
61 Broadway, 6th Floor
New York, NY 10006
Phone: (212) 315-8700
http://www.lungusa.org

A vast resource for education and information; provides a Lung Help Line to answer questions.

American Medical Association
515 N. State Street
Chicago, IL 60610
Phone: (800) 621-8335
http://www.ama-assn.org

The nation's largest physician's group that advocates on issues vital to the nation's health.

Atlanta Medical Center
303 Parkway Drive NE
Atlanta, GA 30312
Phone: (404) 265-4000
http://www.atlantamedcenter.com

A comprehensive cancer care center.

American Society of Clinical Oncology
1900 Duke Street, Suite 200
Alexandria, VA 22314
Phone: (703) 299-0150
http://www.asco.org

International society of cancer specialists; its web site provides resources and patient guides

Brigham and Women's Hospital Center of Excellence: Cancer
75 Francis Street
Boston, MA 02115
Phone: (617) 732-5500
http://www.brighamandwomens.org/excellence/cancer.aspx

Devoted to helping people fight cancer.

Cancer & Careers
http://www.cancerandcareers.org/

Resources for working women with cancer.

Cancer Information Service
1-(800) 4-CANCER
http://cis.nci.nih.gov/

Information center

Cancer Registry
http://data-management.8bestsites.info/data/cancer-registry-data-management.html

Lists top sites for cancer registry.

Cancer Survivor and Wellness Support Group

Bellevue Unity Church
16330 NE 4th Street
Bellevue, WA
Phone: (206) 286-6623
http://www.westayhealthy.com

Seattle-area support group.

Cancer Treatment Centers of America

Phone: (800) 392-9855
http://www.cancercenter.com

Provides information on cancer treatment hospitals and facilities.

Dana-Farber Cancer Institute

44 Binney Street
Boston, MA 02115
Phone: (866) 408-3324
http://www.dfci.harvard.edu

Provides care to children and adults diagnosed with cancer.

Emory University's Woodruff Health Sciences Center

Lung Cancer.org – Lung Cancer 101
Phone: 1-(877) 646-LUNG
http://www.lungcancer.org

Information for patients and care givers.

Environmental Protection Agency

Ariel Rios Building
1200 Pennsylvania Avenue NW
Washington D.C. 20460
Phone (202) 206-2090
http://www.epa.gov

Promotes public health through the environment with links to other resources

Global Lung Cancer Coalition
http://www.lungcancercoalition.org

Promotes global understanding of the burden of lung cancer and patient advocacy.

Hubbard Hospice House in Charleston, WV
1143 Dunbar Avenue
Dunbar, WV 25064
Phone: (304) 768-8523
http://www.kanawhahospice.org/hhtour.html

Specializes in health care services for the terminally ill.

Iaround.org
2400 Chestnut Street, Suite 2908
Philadelphia, PA 19103
http://www.iaround.org/

Lung cancer guide and resources.

Joan's Legacy: The Joan Scarangello Foundation to Conquer Lung Cancer
27 Union Square West, Suite 304
New York, NY 10003
Phone: (212) 627-5500
http://www.joanslegacy.org

Foundation funding innovative research and increasing lung cancer awareness; special focus on non-smoking-related lung cancer.

Johns Hopkins Medical Center
600 North Wolfe Street
Baltimore, Maryland 21287
Phone: (410) 955-5000
http://www.hopkinsmedicine.org

Specializes in the diagnosis and treatment of disease.

Livestrong—The Lance Armstrong Foundation
P.O. Box 161150
Austin, TX 78716-1150
Phone: (512) 236-8820
http://www.livestrong.org

A non-profit organization that inspires and empowers people with cancer.

Lombardi Comprehensive Cancer Center at Georgetown University
3800 Reservoir Road NW
Washington, D.C. 20057
Phone: (202) 444-4000
http://lombardi.georgetown.edu

Provides clinical care, research and education.

Lung Cancer Alliance
888 16th Street, NW, Suite 800
Washington, D.C. 20006
Phone: (202) 463-2080
http://www.lungcanceralliance.org

A national non-profit organization dedicated to lung cancer patient support and advocacy.

Lung Cancer Circle of Hope
7 Carnation Drive, Suite A
Lakewood, NJ 08701
Phone: (732) 363-4426
http://www.lungcancercircleofhope.org

Educates, advocates, and promotes increased funding for lung cancer research.

Lung Cancer Focus Healthology, Inc.
500 Seventh Avenue, 14th Floor
New York, NY 10018
http://www.lungcancerfocus.com/lungcancer/resources.asp

Physician-generated health and medical information.

Lung Cancer Online
http://www.lungcanceronline.org/care/hosploCTors.html
http://www.lungcanceronline.org/sites/pharmcos.html

Hospital and cancer center programs locator; lists pharmaceutical companies.

Lungevity Foundation
2421 N. Ashland Avenue
Chicago, IL 60614
Phone: (773) 281-LUNG
http://www.lungevity.org

Online lung cancer support community and fundraiser for lung cancer research.

Massachusetts General Hospital Pulmonary and Critical Care Unit

55 Fruit Street
Boston, MA 02114
Phone: (617) 726-3735
http://www.mgh.harvard.edu/pulmonary

Provides comprehensive clinical care for pulmonary patients

National Cancer Institute (United States National Institutes of Health)

NCI Public Inquiries Office
6116 Executive Boulevard, Room 3036A
Bethesda, MD 20892-8322
Phone: 1-(800) -4-CANCER
http://www.cancer.gov

Answers questions about cancer and provides information materials.

National Center for Complementary and Alternative Medicine

National Institutes of Health
9000 Rockville Pike
Bethesda, MD 20892
Phone: (301) 496-4000
http://nccam.nih.gov

National Institutes of Health (United States Department of Health & Human Services)

9000 Rockville Pike
Bethesda, Maryland 20892
Phone: (301) 496-4000
http://health.nih.gov

Information about health and diagnosed disorders.

National Lung Cancer Partnership
222 N. Midvale Blvd., Suite 6
Madison, WI 53705
Phone: (608) 233-7905
http://www.nationallungcancerpartnership.org/

Raises awareness and promotes funding for lung cancer research.

New Jersey Commission on Cancer Research
Department of Health and Senior Services
P.O. Box 360
Trenton, NJ 08625-0360
http://www.state.nj.us/health/ccr/njccradvisory.htm

Cancer prevention and control advisory group board.

North Shore-Long Island Jewish Health System
http://www.northshorelij.com

The nation's third largest non-profit secular health care system; provides list of hospitals and facilities including contact information.

OnCoChat
http://www.oncochat.org/oncores.htm

Online peer support for cancer survivors, families, and friends.

OncoLink—Abramson Cancer Center of the University of Pennsylvania
http://ga.elungcancer.net

Resources and information about lung cancer and Mesothelioma.

Research Advocacy Network
309 E. Rand Road, Suite 175
Arlington Heights, IL 60004
Phone: (877) 276-2187
http://www.researchadvocacy.org

A non-profit organization that brings together all interested participants in the medical research process.

Stonybrook University Medical Center
Nicolls Road and Health Sciences Drive Intersection
Stony Brook, NY 11794
http://www.stonybrookmedicalcenter.org

Provides patient care, research, education and community service.

The Princeton Longevity Center
46 Vreeland Drive
Princeton, NJ 08558
Phone: (866) 794-4325
http://www.theplc.net/lungscans.shtml

Lung cancer screening.

University of Massachusetts Memorial Hospital Health Care
Biotech One
365 Plantation Street
Worcester, MA 01605
Phone: (508) 334-1000
http://www.umassmemorial.org/

The largest health care system in Central and Western Massachusetts.